"Dr. Shamsuddin wrote this book to summarize his lifetime research on IP$_6$, so that readers can clearly and easily understand the potential of inositol compounds. Previous to this current work, Dr. Shamsuddin advocated "field effect theory" of colorectal carcinogenesis and invented several new tests for the early detection of colorectal cancer (CRC), one of which is gaining popularity worldwide in screening cancerous and precancerous conditions of CRC. His painstaking research efforts then turned IP$_6$ and its great potential as a chemopreventive and chemotherapeutic agent for cancer. IP$_6$ and inositol compounds now await clinical use for human cancer prevention and therapy. Read this book and learn about the amazing beneficial actions of inositol and IP$_6$."

Kosaku Sakamoto, MD, DMSc
Sakamoto Clinic of Gastroenterology

"Dr. Shamsuddin, who as a pathologist at the University of Maryland sees daily the ravages of cancer, made pioneer observations on the effect of IP$_6$ supported by experiments. This is a challenging and very interesting book on cancer research and treatment."

George Weber, MD
Distinguished Professor and Director
Laboratory for Experimental Oncology
Indiana University School of Medicine

BOOK YOUR PLACE ON OUR WEBSITE AND MAKE THE READING CONNECTION!

We've created a customized website just for our very special readers, where you can get the inside scoop on everything that's going on with Zebra, Pinnacle and Kensington books.

When you come online, you'll have the exciting opportunity to:

- View covers of upcoming books

- Read sample chapters

- Learn about our future publishing schedule (listed by publication month *and author*)

- Find out when your favorite authors will be visiting a city near you

- Search for and order backlist books from our online catalog

- Check out author bios and background information

- Send e-mail to your favorite authors

- Meet the Kensington staff online

- Join us in weekly chats with authors, readers and other guests

- Get writing guidelines

- AND MUCH MORE!

**Visit our website at
http://www.kensingtonbooks.com**

IP$_6$

NATURE'S REVOLUTIONARY CANCER-FIGHTER

AbulKalam M. Shamsuddin, MD, PhD

Kensington Books
http://www.kensingtonbooks.com

NOTE TO READER

This book represents a wealth of scientific information gained through numerous experiments and studies. Although there may be sections where technical terminology is necessary, the author has attempted to express his ideas in as nontechnical a manner as possible.

To my fellow human beings suffering from cancer . . .
May this humble effort help alleviate your pain.

Contents

Acknowledgments 11
Introduction: IP_6: Nature's Sweet Gift 13

CHAPTER 1. The Fiber Connection 19
  Fiber: Fad or Fact of Life? 19
  Are All Fibers Created Equal? 23
  "Phyting" Cancer 26

CHAPTER 2. IP_6: What Is It? 28
  IP_6: What's in a Name? 28
  Every Cell In Your Body 29
  Reaping the Harvest 31
  Phytate: Friend or Foe? 34

CHAPTER 3. IP_6 or Fiber: Which Works Best? 37
  Mammary Cancer Studies 37
  Stages of Cancer 39

CHAPTER 4. IP_6: How Does It Protect Us? 45
  It's in the Genes: Protecting Your DNA 45
  Antioxidant Protection: Iron Is Out 47

CHAPTER 5. IP_6: Action Against Cancer 52
  The Cancer Problem 52
  Cancer Prevention 54
  How Does IP_6 Work? 62

CHAPTER 6. Cancer Therapy and IP$_6$ 66
Treating Cancer Cells 66
Which Cancers Could Be Treated by IP$_6$? 72
Boosting Natural Killers 76

CHAPTER 7. Other Benefits of IP$_6$ 79
Inflammation and Fibrosis 79
Kidney Stones 80
Heart Disease 83
Heart Attack 85
*Blood Benefits: More Oxygen and Less Sickle Cell
    Anemia 87*
Cholesterol and Triglycerides 88

CHAPTER 8. And That's Not All 90
Defusing Liver Cancer Cells 90
*Rhabdomyosarcoma: A Malignant Childhood
    Cancer 92*
Colon Cancer: IP$_6$ vs. Green Tea 97
Safety of IP$_6$ 99

CHAPTER 9. Inositol: Mother of IP$_6$ 104
A Unique B Vitamin 104
Health Benefits of Inositol 108

**CHAPTER 10. An Anticancer Cocktail: IP$_6$ +
            Inositol 115**
Making a Good Thing Better 115
Cancer-Fighting Combination 117
How Much to Take? 121

Epilogue 122
*On the Horizon: Increasing p53, a Tumor
    Suppressor 123*

The World Takes Notice 124
Best of Both Worlds 127

References 128
Resources 141
About the Author 143

ACKNOWLEDGMENTS

All new scientific breakthroughs follow a pathway before the facts reach the public. First there is discovery and an idea or hypothesis about how this new idea can be put to use. This is followed by a long period of experimenting and testing to prove the hypothesis. Results of studies must be published, and colleagues and institutions must be convinced of the benefits and safety of a new method or substance. My discovery of the anticancer function of IP_6 + inositol followed such a pathway. The road was often rocky, but my vision of bringing this vital information to those who could most benefit was a motivating force. It has been said of science and medicine that old ideas take 50 years to be replaced while new ideas take 100 years to reach acceptance. Thank goodness the wait is over and the knowledge is now in your hands. To accomplish this journey successfully, I needed help.

Fortunately, my friends and supporters worked tirelessly, and selflessly—some even worked without financial remuneration. These are true examples of dedication. For that I am indebted to them, especially to my friend and associate Dr. Ivana Vucenik, who for nearly a decade has been the backbone of the IP_6 project. Dr. Kosaku Sakamoto of Gunma University, Japan, believed in this work enough to give up his successful practice of surgery for 2 years to work with me on IP_6. I am also indebted to my friend Dr. Maryce Jacobs, former Vice-President of Research at the American Institute for Cancer Research (AIRC); without her support and AICR's grants, I couldn't have done many of the experiments.

I wish also to thank medical writer Jean Barilla, M.S., for her help in putting this book together and Lee Heiman, my editor at Kensington Publishing, for making it possible to present this valuable information to you, the reader.

And finally, even the best discovery or invention has no value unless it's being used. Thus my gratitude to Terry Lemerond and Matthew Schueller of Enzymatic Therapy for bringing the fruit of this discovery to the benefit of mankind.

IP$_6$: Nature's Sweet Gift

One of nature's most important gifts for the preservation of health and life itself is inositol, considered a member of the B complex family of vitamins. Inositol is found in almost every cell and is essential for key body functions. The brain, the nervous system, and the reproductive organs all depend on a constant supply of inositol. Most importantly, in relation to cancer, inositol helps control the growth and number of cells. Cancerous cells arise in our bodies every day, but our immune system can usually keep these invaders in check. When cells multiply without control, they can overwhelm the body's immune system, and cancer can take hold. Inositol and its family of related molecules, the inositol phosphates, work in concert to prevent such an event.

Inositol is similar in its chemical structure to glucose and is thus called a "sugar." While it does have a sweet taste, that is the least of its abilities. Small changes in its chemical structure—such as the addition of phosphate groups (PO$_4$—an atom of the mineral phosphorus [P] plus four oxygen atoms [O])—produce a whole family of inositol phosphates, each with its own repertoire of biochemical effects in the body. Figure 1 shows a simplified chemical structure for inositol hexaphosphate—inositol + 6 phosphate groups.

**Figure 1. Chemical structure of
Inositol hexaphosphate (phytic acid)**

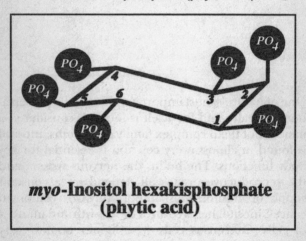

***myo*-Inositol hexakisphosphate
(phytic acid)**

Chemical structure of inositol hexaphosphate. It is a ring structure, with the lines between the numbers representing bonds between atoms of carbon. The numbers 1–6 represent the location of carbon atoms where phosphate groups (PO$_4$) are attached on the structure. P = phosphorus; O = oxygen.

There are six places on inositol for phosphate to attach, so the phosphate derivatives are named according to the number of phosphate groups attached: inositol monophosphate (IP$_1$), inositol biphosphate

(IP_2), inositol triphosphate (IP_3), and so on through IP_4 and IP_5. When all 6 phosphate groups are attached, the molecule is called inositol hexaphosphate (or IP_6, sometimes called $InsP_6$, and previously called phytic acid). IP_6 can revert to inositol by losing phosphate groups, and inositol can be converted back to IP_6 by gaining phosphate groups. IP_6 and inositol are synergistic: the health effects of the combination are greater than that of each form alone. As we will see, this addition of inositol to IP_6 makes it an even better *anticancer cocktail.*

Pioneering experiments done in my laboratory have shown that IP_6 causes a consistent, reproducible and statistically significant reduction in cancers that affect various tissues and organs including the colon, breast, prostate, and liver. Scientists around the world are also confirming, validating, and expanding on this work.

When a study is *statistically significant,* it has produced results that will be accepted as valid by all researchers. A study may show an effect of a treatment, but not have a large enough number of patients in the study for the results to be "statistically significant." In this case, study results will not be accepted by scientists, conventional medical practitioners, or the more discerning practitioners of complementary or alternative medicine.

We are only beginning to understand the value of some of these inositol compounds in the life process. We know that inositol is an essential nutrient for cells to survive in the laboratory; virtually every single cell type that one wishes to grow (or "culture") must be supplied with inositol. In laboratory and animal experiments, inositol has demonstrated striking properties in the prevention and treatment of cancer. The inositol phosphates in red blood cells may play a very important role in regulating their oxygen-carrying capacity. This role may have relevance in the treatment of sickle cell anemia.

Work done mostly by other researchers worldwide and published in highly respected professional peer-reviewed journals show that *in addition to being an anticancer agent, IP$_6$ is also an antioxidant.* It can reverse the effect of the damaging free radicals produced during oxidation reactions in the body, as we will see in later chapters. IP$_6$ prevents kidney stone formation and fatty liver. It can also increase the body's resistance to infection. IP$_6$ acts to reduce two key risk factors for heart disease: serum cholesterol and triglycerides. It also prevents damage to the heart muscle cells during a heart attack. Inositol has been used in treatment of psychiatric disorders, and has been shown to be effective in preventing many of the complications associated with diabetes mellitus. We even know that the seeds of certain plants may remain viable (alive and able to grow) for 400 years; one reason for such longevity may be IP$_6$. As our knowledge and understanding improves, we find more and more of these inositol derivatives to be interesting and perhaps crucial to all life—humans, animals, and plants.

IP$_6$ is a unique compound and has been my favorite among the inositol molecules. If one said that IP$_6$ will be the aspirin of the twenty-first century, it would not be totally inaccurate, except that it is much better, because its use and potential for use is far greater than aspirin, and it is much safer too.

I believe that IP_6 has the potential to surpass what is already known of its health benefits! This book is my way of sharing with you a gift that nature has provided.

Where can you find this inositol and IP_6? Inositol hexaphosphate (IP_6) and inositol are commonly found in cereals and legumes. Because these nutrients are abundant in high-fiber diets, this may explain, at least in part, the finding that high-fiber diets are associated with a lower incidence of certain cancers. So to set the stage for the role of IP_6 and inositol as a cancer fighter, let's first talk about fiber.

CHAPTER 1

The Fiber Connection

Fiber: Fad or Fact of Life?

Fiber has been in and out of the media spotlight for the past two decades. First we hear that it is good for us, then just how good becomes a topic of debate. "Insoluble fiber like wheat bran sweeps the intestines like a broom." "Oat bran, a soluble fiber, gets cholesterol out of the body." "Fiber fights cancer." "Fiber may fight cancer." "Fiber is not so important in fighting cancer." So many statements—too many opinions. So what are the key facts on fiber that you need to know?

Dietary fibers are found in the plants we eat. The fibers are resistant to digestion by our digestive enzymes or by the enzymes produced by the intestinal flora. Flora refers to the population of helpful microorganisms that live in our bodies in places such as the colon and on the skin surfaces of our bodies. These are the bacteria that live with us and do work in return for room and board. It is estimated that we have about three pounds of intestinal bacteria in our bodies; without it we would die. Depending on how resistant to digestion a fiber is, it is called soluble (less resistant) or insoluble (very resistant).

We have heard that fibers are good for us because they increase the stool bulk. This is a step in the right direction toward normal elimination. But do all fibers increase stool bulk? Since the soluble fibers are broken down (degraded) in the intestine, they increase stool bulk only moderately. Insoluble fibers, on the other hand, absorb a lot of water and thus greatly increase the stool size.

The major components of fiber are polysaccharides, which is another name for carbohydrates. All carbohydrates contain carbon, hydrogen, and oxygen with these atoms arranged in different ways to form the various types in the group. This group includes cellulose, hemicellulose, pectins, gums, mucilages, and lignin. Chemically speaking, soluble fibers (pectins, gums, mucilages, and some hemicellulose molecules) can be partially digested in the intestinal tract. The insoluble fibers (lignin, cellulose, and some hemicellulose molecules), however, are poorly degraded in the gut. So for ability to increase the bulk of stool, insoluble fibers are the natural choice.

Which type of foods have soluble and insoluble fibers? Soluble fibers are present in fruits and vegetables and some grains such as oats. While fruits and vegetables contain some insoluble fibers, cereals, particularly whole grain cereals, are our major source of insoluble fiber. And it is the outer coatings of cereal grains, the bran part, that is rich in insoluble fiber.

We consume fibers in different forms. For example, our diet includes fiber as whole foods—whole cereal grains, legumes (beans and peas), fruits, and vegetables. We also take in fiber-rich additions to our diet—brans from wheat, corn, and rice. Isolated and purified fiber components such as cellulose, pectins, gums, and lignin are also added to our foods. Or we take them individually for specific reasons. For example, the husk from the seeds of a kind of plantain, *Plantago ovata,* and its close relative, psyllium seeds, *Plantago psyllium,* have been used as laxatives because of their strong water-absorbing, or hydrophilic, properties.

The usefulness of fiber in health has been recognized for some time. Initially there is the work of Dr. George Oettle of South Africa. Further developments by Dr. Dennis Burkitt, who is generally credited for advocating the benefits of dietary fiber in prevention of colon cancer, were very important here. In 1968, however, at least four years prior to Dr. Burkitt, another researcher from India, Dr. S. L. Malhotra, published information on the colon cancer connection. Even if one takes in to account Dr. Burkitt's reference to the health benefits of fiber in the journal *Lancet* in 1969, Dr. Malhotra clearly precedes him by a year.

The dietary habits in India vary from region to region as well as among different religious groups. From an extensive study of the food habits between north and south Indian populations, Dr. Malhotra was the first to conclusively demonstrate that people who eat a high-fiber diet are at a reduced risk of various diseases, including colon cancer. He observed that cancer of the colon was far less common in north India as compared to the south. He explained, ''While the north Indian diets are rich in roughage, cellulose, and vegetable fibers, these are almost completely lacking in the south Indian diets.''

How does fiber act to inhibit colon cancer? Fiber can dilute or absorb (stick to) cancer-causing substances (carcinogens) or cancer-promoting chemicals in the gut. It can also cause a faster transit time for the stool. In this respect it acts like a broom, sweeping out the intestinal debris. Not paying attention to these housekeeping duties can result in such problems as diverticulitis. This condition is an inflammation of a diverticulum, the small pockets in the wall of the colon which fill with stagnant stool. Having a number of these pockets is called diverticulosis and it is common in middle age. Inflammation of these pockets can cause discomfort and pain, and more rarely, they may cause obstruction, perforation, or bleeding. When the stool exits faster, there is also less opportunity for the cancer-promoting and cancer-causing agents in the dietary remains to interact with intestinal cells.

Even though Dr. Malhotra presented and published the first scientific evidence, thanks go to Dr. Burkitt, who propagated and popularized the concept that fiber is beneficial to our health through many repeated lectures and publications. His lectures especially were accompanied by slides showing the beneficial effects of fiber on the intestinal contents. And for nearly three decades thereafter, eating a high-fiber diet remained popular. Unfortunately, the scientific community, and therefore the government and private agencies that give research grants, have quietly abandoned fiber. Why? The complete answer is unclear. But it may be because fiber, as you have had a slight glimpse, is a complex substance. It contains many nutrients. Rice bran, for example, contains protein, healthy oil, vitamins (such as vitamin E), antioxidants (i.e., gamma-oryzanol), lecithin, and of course, inositol and its family of phosphate-containing molecules. When carbohydrates are metabolized in the body, many such as inositol will end up containing phosphorus, the atom found in the phosphate group. Other types of bran have nutrients in common with rice bran, but have more or less of other different components. Trying to decide which substance is doing what function in the body is not an easy task!

Interest in fiber was further decreased after research began to indicate that a high-fat intake was associated with a high risk of breast and other cancers. So all eyes turned to investigating the effects of fat in the diet, and fiber research was neglected.

If you think about it, though, isn't it true that eating a high-fat and high-protein diet automatically lowers the intake of fiber? For many people, a nice juicy steak or two eggs with bacon and sausage are more appealing than a bowl of salad or beans! And when you are planning to have a filet mignon, you tend to cut down on the bread, salad, and side vegetables, so that you can enjoy that steak. So as we reduce the intake of fiber and increase the intake of fat and protein in our diet, we lose something; the health benefits clearly associated with fiber. It just may be that the reduction in fiber, rather than the increase in fat, contributes more to colon cancer.

Are All Fibers Created Equal?

When cells divide, it is a time when the genetic material (the DNA) is duplicated. At this time the

genes in the nucleus of the cell uncoil. Then the
DNA double strands that make up the gene unwind.
This open structure is needed for copies to be made
of each DNA strand. Once the copies are made, each
resulting set of doubled DNA will end up in a new
"daughter" cell. When the DNA is in an opened
structure, it is especially vulnerable to attack by cancer-
causing agents. Increasing the rate of cell division
therefore increases the risk of attack. Whenever DNA
is being copied, there is also a greater risk of inaccurate copying taking place. So increasing the amount
of cell division allows more "mistakes" or mutations
to happen, and more damage to occur when the
DNA is copied. Increased cell division is a first step
toward getting cancer. Exposing cells or animals to
agents that increase cell division is a way to enhance
the incidence of experimental cancers in the laboratory. Experimental studies in rodents, for instance,
have shown that certain high-fiber diets can actually
increase cell division in the colon.

As I said before, fiber is a complicated substance—
its effects can vary depending on other dietary factors.
Dr. Lucien R. Jacobs at the University of California,
Davis, showed that oat bran and corn bran actually
increased experimentally produced colon cancer in
rats. According to Dr. Jacobs, the reason for the
increase was that a high-fiber oat and corn diet
increased the acidity level of the colon. When these
fibers are broken down by the microbes in the bowel,
fatty acids are produced. These fatty acids are used
as fuel by the cells lining the intestine. The energy
that the cells get from this fuel is known to cause the
cells to divide and proliferate. The oat bran in the
rats' diet represented 20% of the total diet—a large
amount. To make up for the reduced calories in the

high-fiber diet, the rats ate more food. Eating more is another factor that may have affected the health of the rats. Studies with corn bran also found significantly more colon tumors at high levels (20%) of bran in the diet. There was a reduction, however, in tumor number when the rats were fed diets with lower levels (4.5% of the diet). When rice and soybean brans were fed at a 20% level, even with high fat in the diet, there were no significant effects on tumor incidence. Although the researchers stated that the results were difficult to compare with other studies because of the varying amounts of fiber and fat, the experimental studies do show that the *types of* fiber are important.

Large-scale studies on the occurrence and distribution of cancer in the population have been done by several groups of researchers. They investigated the relationship between fiber and diseases, and the type of high-fiber food and cancer. Dr. David G. Zaridze, for one, discussed these complex interactions in an article in the *Journal of the National Cancer Institute* (1983). He said that dietary factors are now considered to be one of the most important risk factors for cancer, ranking at least second after tobacco. According to Dr. Zaridze, large-bowel or colon cancer is one of the most strongly related to the diet. He also discussed three studies that showed a possible protective effect of high fiber intake. In one study cancer patients were found to have eaten significantly less amounts of fiber less frequently. In another study, more cancer patients than study subjects without cancer ate diets high in saturated fat–rich food and low in fiber-rich foods. In a Japanese study, a higher daily intake of rice and wheat was associated with fewer deaths from colon and rectal cancers. It turns out though that not all high-fiber diets are correlated with a reduced incidence of, for instance, colon cancer. The only high-fiber diets that are strongly and consistently associated with a low incidence of colon cancer are those from cereals, particularly rice and wheat. So what makes cereals different from other high-fiber diets?

"Phyting" Cancer

Cereals and legumes (beans, peas) as you know by now, have more of the insoluble type of fiber, particularly in the outer bran layer. The bran contains that very important "sugar," inositol hexaphosphate (IP$_6$), also called phytic acid or phytate. Calling it phytic acid gives the impression that it is similar to acids such as nitric acid or sulfuric acid. There are many acids, however, that are beneficial to health (i.e., folic acid, the B vitamin). The word "acid" just refers to the chemical structure and does not indicate the degree of "acidity."

Phytate is naturally found in most cereals, nuts, legumes, and oil seeds in amounts ranging from 1% to 5% of the plant. In addition to acting as an antioxidant (as explained in Chapter 4), phytate can protect cells from harmful reactions. For example, the mineral iron, although necessary for the function of red blood cells, can be damaging in excess amounts. Phytate can prevent the excess iron from interacting with and damaging the cells. Phytate can do this by surrounding and shielding, or chelating, iron atoms. In chemical terms, chelating describes the ability of a molecule such as phytate to surround an iron atom, effectively shielding it from interaction with other cellular structures. Phytate has a high affinity for iron, chelating it and preventing it from reaction with oxygen. When iron reacts with oxygen, very reactive molecules called free radicals are formed. Phytate is acting as an antioxidant in this case, because it has inactivated the oxidant (iron).

Dr. Ernst Graf and his associate John Eaton, who were researchers working at the Pillsbury Company, in an editorial in the journal *Cancer* (1985), questioned whether our health benefits are due to fiber or phytate. Dr. Graf discussed a study on the effects of fiber. In the study, the dietary habits of people in Finland showed that the Finnish population eats a more cereal-based diet. They thereby consume more phytate, as opposed to the Danes who have less phytate in their diet, even though their total fiber intake is double that of the Finns. Surprisingly, the Finns have half the incidence of colon cancer than the Danes do! Thus, Danes who eat double the amount of fiber have twice as much cancer! Drs. Graf and Eaton thus proposed that perhaps it is the high phytate in the Finnish diet and the low amount in the Danish diet that can explain this phenomenon.

CHAPTER 2

IP$_6$: What Is It?

IP$_6$: What's in a Name?

It was a Saturday afternoon in the summer of 1985. I remember taking the August 15 issue of the journal *Cancer* out of my mailbox, going through its table of contents as I was walking back to the house . . . and I saw the provocative title "Dietary Suppression of Colonic Cancer: Fiber or Phytate?" by Dr. Ernst Graf (whose work I discussed in Chapter 1). Thanks to Dr. Graf, I became acquainted with phytate. Needless to say, I was fascinated. As I was reading and rereading the article, it dawned on me that the phytate Dr. Graf was talking about was one of the six different inositol phosphates in the cell.

This was the era when researchers were starting to investigate the inositol phosphates. Inositol *tri*-phosphate (IP$_3$) had been found to be a key molecule in conveying chemical information within the cell. In keeping with the naming process, I thought: Why not call it inositol hexaphosphate, or IP_6 for short; since this name would indicate that it was part of the bigger family of inositol compounds. Thinking of it in this way allowed me to formulate some hypotheses and devise experiments for the following years, culminating in discovery of many health benefits of this unique compound.

Every Cell in Your Body

Inositol hexaphosphate (abbreviated as IP_6, and also known as phytic acid or phytate) was first identified in 1855. It is found in almost all mammalian cells, including human cells, where it is necessary in regulating vital cellular functions. Its concentration is high in heart muscle, brain, and skeletal muscle. Cell membranes protect all cells and allow nutrients in and cell products (including waste products) out of the cell. These membranes contain special molecules called phospholipids. Phospholipids are made of essential fats and the mineral phosphorus. Phosphatidylinositol is one of these phospholipids. When hormones, neurotransmitters, and other chemical substances in the body interact with cell membranes, inositol breaks off with various numbers of phosphorus groups attached. These are the inositol phosphates, including IP_6 (inositol hexaphosphate, as described in Chapter 1). Another inositol phosphate, IP_3, is known to affect calcium metabolism in cells. Understanding what these inositol phosphates do in the body is a key project for researchers. And as you might guess by now, IP$_6$ is proving to be an exciting molecule with many health applications.

Biochemists and cell biologists have been interested in a curious process that happens to IP$_6$. In this process, phosphate groups can be added to (phosphorylation) or may come off (dephosphorylation) the inositol. From one to six of these phosphate groups can be present. (See the Introduction, Figure 1.) The interest is in how this process might affect the way cells work. Lower inositol phosphates (IP$_1$, IP$_2$, IP$_3$, and IP$_4$) are known to carry messages between cells. When one of these IP molecules touches a molecule or cell structure, it transmits a chemical "message." And this is done in one of two ways. Either the IPs can bind to the outside of cell membranes that surround cells and cause events to occur inside them, or they can act inside of cells directly.

The messenger role of inositol 1,4,5-tri-phosphate (IP$_3$) in bringing about a host of cellular functions is well recognized. The numbers in front of the name here correspond to the carbon atoms on inositol to which the phosphate groups are attached. There are six carbon atoms altogether in inositol. These functions of IP$_3$ include starting cell division (mitosis) by releasing calcium stored in the cell. Its cousin, 1,3,4,5-tetraphosphate (IP$_4$), has been shown to cause calcium to be stored in the cell. Higher forms of inositol phosphates, inositol 1,3,4,5,6-pentaphosphate (IP$_5$) and inositol hexaphosphate (IP$_6$), are also abundant and represent the bulk of the inositol phosphate content of mammalian cells. IP$_5$ and IP$_6$ are present in virtually all mammalian cells, including human cells, in substantial amounts much higher than any other inositol phosphates. Why should there be an abundance of these compounds in the cell? Nature always has a purpose for everything she does. It may not be immediately obvious, but eventually we discover what biological molecules do in the body.

Recent studies are giving us an increased understanding of how IP$_5$ and IP$_6$ function. For instance, we know that IP$_5$ can regulate the ability of avian (bird) hemoglobin in red blood cells to pick up and hold oxygen. Along with IP$_6$, IP$_5$ may be involved in causing the excitation or stimulation of nerve cells as shown by Dr. Menniti and colleagues (1993). Recent studies also show that IP$_5$ and IP$_6$ are not inactive or "metabolically lethargic" and that they play a more dynamic role in the cell than has previously been appreciated. As described below, one aspect of IP$_6$ receiving increased attention is its role in prevention or in treating cancer.

Reaping the Harvest

As we've discussed, IP$_6$ is found in a variety of places. It is found in plants, and other related substances in the soil, especially the inositol hexaphosphates. IP$_6$ is found in substantial amounts (from 0.4 to 6.4%) in cereals and legumes (peas, beans). Mature soybean seeds contain up to 2.58% of IP$_6$, whereas various soy-based compounds contain much smaller amounts as reported by Drs. Harland and Oberleas in the *World Review of Nutrition and Diet* (1987).

But where exactly is the IP$_6$? IP$_6$ can exist in different parts of seeds depending on the types of seeds.

Table 1.
IP$_6$ Content in Various Seeds

Food	IP$_6$ Content, %
Corn	0–6.4
Sesame	5.3
Wheat	1.1–4.8
Beans	2.5
Rice	2.2
Peanuts	1.9
Sunflower	1.9
Soybeans	0.1–1.8
Textured soy concentrate	1.5
Barley	1.0
Peas	0.9
Oats	0.8

For example, in rice and wheat seeds—which are part of the monocotyledonous seed family—IP$_6$ accumulates in the particles that make up the bran (or aleurone) layer. Now the name *cotyledon* refers to the first single leaf that sprouts from the seed. With castor, peanut, cotton seeds, and beans—which are part of the dicotyledonous seed family—two seed leaves sprout, not one. The different family names, of course, are used to classify different types of plants. And in dicotyledonous seeds IP$_6$ is found within the seed as phytin—an arrangement where IP$_6$ is found together with potassium and magnesium (called a "salt" of IP$_6$). Figure 2 shows an aleurone particle isolated from a rice grain. It contains several phytin inclusions.

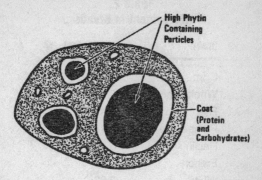

Figure 2. Schematic diagram of the presence of IP_6 (as phytin) in an aleurone particle. From Ogawa, Tanaka, and Kasai (1975).

Because IP_6 is concentrated in the bran (outer layers of the seeds) in cereals such as rice, wheat, and rye, normal milling or processing which removes bran, also reduces the total IP_6 content of the seeds. Polished (white) rice, for instance, a fad of the recent decades is, therefore, deficient in IP_6. For its part, corn is different from other grains in that most of its IP_6 content, about 88%, is concentrated in the germ portion of the kernel. In this case, "degermed" corn would be deficient in IP_6. The IP_6 content in various breads is shown in Table 2.

Regard for IP_6 has had its ups and downs, like a roller-coaster ride, ever since its discovery. Its early popularity stemmed mostly from the fact that it is the chief storage form of phosphorous, a necessary nutrient for germinating seeds and for all cells. Phosphorous is a key part of a very important (probably the most important) molecule in all cells: ATP. ATP, or adenosine triphosphate, is the molecule that stores

Table 2.
IP$_6$ Content in Breads

Bread	IP$_6$ Content, %
Corn	1.36
Whole wheat	0.56
Rye	0.41
Pumpernickel	0.16
Raisin	0.09
French	0.03
White	0.03

energy in every cell. Without it, cells would cease to function, and the organism of which these cells are made would die. This is true for plants, animals, and anything that is alive. So in addition to its anticancer action, IP$_6$ is supplying phosphorus, a critical energy ingredient. Other interest in IP$_6$ is due to its antioxidant function, which I will discuss in Chapter 4.

Phytate: Friend or Foe?

The "good press" given to IP$_6$, however, has sometimes been ignored because of a misunderstanding of its role in mineral metabolism. During the past half century some researchers have discussed the possibility of a mineral deficiency resulting from the intake of foods high in phytate. Our health-conscious society has lately switched from a meat and potato type diet to a more plant-based diet which is high in fiber and phytate and this move has renewed interest in phytate. Food products that not only look and smell but also taste like meat have been developed from soybeans. Consequently, they contain appreciable amounts of IP_6. This topic needs some additional explanation.

One of the things that IP_6 does is to form tight complexes (or chelates) with a variety of nutritionally important minerals, from calcium to zinc. The word *chelate* comes from the Greek word for "claw." The mineral is held inside a claw or basket-like structure made up of the IP_6 molecule, hence the name.

More specifically, *in vitro* (in the laboratory) IP_6 forms complexes with certain mineral atoms, each positively charged and known as ions. In decreasing order of chelating ability these mineral atoms are copper (Cu), zinc (Zn), cobalt (Co), manganese (Mn), iron (Fe), and calcium (Ca). It was commonly thought that IP_6 reduced the bioavailability of these dietary minerals; that is, chelating keeps the minerals from being used in the body. So most interest thus far has been focused on the potential inhibitory effect of IP_6 on mineral absorption.

But is this focus valid?

The usual scientific procedure in trying to determine the properties of a substance is for it to be evaluated in its pure form (or as pure as it can be obtained). Most, if not all, of the studies reporting that IP_6 inhibits, for example, iron absorption, have not been done on its pure form. Rather, these studies have been done on diets that are rich in food sources of IP_6. Absent here is the pure or isolated compound. Now it is known that IP_6 contained in food also binds to proteins in food, making it susceptible to destruction by intestinal enzymes. There is much less of it to act on against cancer or other diseases. Protein binding also slows IP_6 absorption from the stomach. It is thus present for a longer time in an area where it can interact with minerals. Pure IP$_6$ is involved in much less protein binding, making it available to cells more quickly and in larger amounts. As we will see in Chapter 8, mineral chelation is really not a problem with IP$_6$ or with phytate consumption.

CHAPTER 3

IP$_6$ or Fiber: Which Works Best?

One component of insoluble fiber, phytic acid (IP$_6$), has proven to be particularly effective in preventing colon cancer induction in models.

—J.H. Weisburger et al. (1993)

Mammary Cancer Studies

We now know that IP$_6$ is more effective against cancer than high fiber. To understand why, we can look at an experiment that was designed to determine which nutrient is more effective in inhibiting rat mammary (breast) cancer.

While most of the studies of diet and breast cancer have been focused on the role of fat, very few have looked at the effect of fiber. Population studies and laboratory research suggest that a typical diet in the Western world, with a high intake of dietary fat and calories and low intake of dietary fiber, increases the risk for breast cancers. It has been difficult to interpret this information. High-fat diets are generally low in fiber content, and it is not clear whether an increased cancer incidence is associated with the harmful effects of fat or with the lack of a beneficial effect of fiber, or both. An interesting exception is the typical Finnish diet, which is high in fat and in fiber. Surprisingly, the breast cancer mortality (death) rate is considerably lower in Finland than in the United States, as reported by Dr. D. P. Rose in 1992, and by Dr. H. Adlercreutz and colleagues in 1994. In other studies investigating the differences in diet-related factors for breast cancer among white, Hispanic, and black college students in New York City, Dr. Zang and his colleagues (1994) found some important differences. The white students were at higher risk than their Hispanic or black classmates. This was, in part, a reflection of the protective agents present in greater amounts in the diets of Hispanic students (beans) and black students (fruits and vegetables) than in the diets of white students. This and other recent studies by Drs. De Stefani and colleagues (1997), Dunn (1994), and Drs. Kliewer and Smith (1995) point toward the role of dietary factors, other than fat, in affecting the risk for breast cancer.

Since we knew that eating whole-grain cereal lowers the risk of intestinal diseases such as appendicitis and colon cancer, we decided to see if there was an effect on breast cancer. We also knew that IP$_6$ is particularly abundant in the bran part of certain mature seeds such as wheat. Earlier studies had shown that pure IP$_6$ (without the bran) was a potent anti-cancer agent that could inhibit cancer. It can even do so at the early stages before cancer is detectable. Before we discuss further studies, however, we need to understand some of the cancer terminology and discuss the stages of cancer.

Stages of Cancer

A tumor can be noncancerous (benign), or it can be cancerous (malignant). The word *cancer* probably comes from the Latin word for "crab" because a cancer "adheres to any part that it seizes upon in an obstinate manner like the crab." Cancer does not just pop into existence overnight. There is a complex interaction between genetics or hereditary and environmental factors such as exposure to toxic substances. Such substances include chemicals, radiation (from the sun and man-made sources), and viruses. Diet plays a large part in influencing the outcome of the interactions between all these factors.

There is a series of steps that occur before a cancer takes hold and overwhelms the body's defenses. When it is a chemical that causes a cancer (as is done experimentally in the laboratory or from environmental exposure), there are two main stages: initiation and promotion. The chemical is the initiator. It causes changes in the cells that make it likely to become cancerous—but initiation alone will not produce cancer. The chemical will only cause permanent damage to the genetic material (the DNA) of the cell. A promoter is needed before the altered cell will become cancerous. The promotor can be another chemical or it could be radiation (X-ray or UV from the sun), or it could be a virus. By itself, of course, the promotor can't cause cancer, but with the initiator damage, it may do so.

A promotor does not have to be there right after

initiation—that is why some cancers take years to develop. An example is exposure to asbestos (an initiator) which is more likely to result in lung cancer years later if a person smokes (the promoter). The fact that cancer does not arise every time a person is exposed to an initiator and subsequently a promotor depends on the strength of the immune system and on how well DNA repair mechanisms work in the body. We make enzymes that will cut away damaged DNA and allow the cell to heal. Making these enzymes depends to a large extent on the raw material supplied from our diet that will be used to make them. Enzymes consist of protein and use vitamins and minerals as cofactors that help the enzymes to function properly. So now that we understand the cancer scenario, we can go back to the studies designed to stop cancer in its tracks.

The study done in my laboratory investigated whether a high-fiber (bran) diet, containing high levels of IP$_6$, would show inhibition, specifically "dose response inhibition," of mammary cancer in rats. Dose response inhibition simply means that a certain dose or amount of a test substance (in this case the bran) would correspond to a certain amount of inhibition of the cancer. Usually, the more test substance given, the more inhibition there is—up to a point. Rats were given three levels of a high-fiber diet (either 5%, 10%, or 20% bran), starting two weeks before carcinogen administration. The carcinogen used throughout the experiment was 7,12-dimethyl-benz[a] anthracene (DMBA). To test whether cereal bran rich in IP$_6$ had the same protective effect as purified IP$_6$ alone, a separate group of rats received the control diet only (the same food without the bran), but IP$_6$ was added in drinking water. Enough

IP_6 was added to equal the content found in the highest bran group. This group received 0.4% IP_6 given in drinking water, which is about equal to the IP_6 content in the 20% bran diet. This amount of IP_6 in the drinking water corresponds to about 500 milligrams to 1000 milligrams of IP_6 if taken in tablets by a 150-pound human. After carcinogen administration, the rats remained on these diets for 29 weeks.

At 29 weeks we found that the rats fed 5%, 10%, and 20% bran had 16.7%, 14.6% and 11.4% reductions of tumor incidence, respectively. These differences are not statistically significant. This means that there was not enough difference compared to the rats who got no bran to be able to tell if the bran was really reducing the incidence of cancer. To be statistically significant, results have to fit certain mathematical formulas that are accepted by all scientists. However, rats given 0.4% IP_6 in drinking water, equal to the amount of IP_6 in 20% bran (or 500 to 1000 milligrams for a human, as noted above), had a 33.5% reduction in tumor incidence and 48.8% fewer tumors per animal—and these numbers *were* significant. The study shows that supplemental dietary fiber in the form of bran had a very modest inhibitory effect, which was not statistically significant. There was no dose-dependent response; in other words, giving more bran did not cause more inhibition of cancer.

In contrast, animals given IP_6 in water (which would be equivalent to about 500 milligrams to 1000 milligrams in a human) showed a significant reduction in tumor number, incidence, and multiplicity (number of tumors per rat). The number of tumors that could be felt by touch (palpable tumors) was 73 in the control group that received no IP_6 or bran.

In the IP$_6$ group, however, the number of palpable tumors was 31. This was a statistically significant 57.2% reduction in tumors for those animals given pure IP$_6$ in their drinking water. Pure IP$_6$ was also highly effective in reducing the multiplication of tumors: there were more tumors per animal in those that got the carcinogen alone or those that just received fiber when compared to the IP$_6$-treated group. Rats that got DMBA and pure IP$_6$ along with their diet did get tumors (see Table 3). The majority of these rats (90%), however, had only 1–2 tumors. For those that received DMBA alone, 45% had 3 or more tumors. In the bran group, 25–42% had 3 or more tumors. This shows that only IP$_6$ in pure form reduced the number of tumors per animal. In four control animals that did not get carcinogen treatment (or any bran or IP$_6$,) there were palpable tumors which were confirmed to be noncancerous or benign (fibroadenomas) tumors. These spontaneously appearing tumors were also found in 2 out of 10 animals receiving the high-fiber diet, but none of the rats in the IP$_6$ group got these tumors. As in our previous experiments, IP$_6$ had also protected the rats against spontaneously appearing mammary tumors.

As shown in Table 3, compared to the group that received only the carcinogen DMBA, only the group getting 0.4% IP$_6$ in drinking water had a significantly reduced tumor incidence. The reduction in the number of rats having 3 or more tumors per rat was also statistically significant. Note that when the rats ate a 20% bran diet containing the same amount (0.4%) of IP$_6$ as the rats receiving pure IP$_6$, it did not reduce any of these cancer factors significantly.

From these results, one conclusion is clear: IP$_6$ is most effective when taken independently of other

Table 3.
Comparison of Bran vs. IP_6

Treatment/Diet Group	Tumor Incidence, %	No. of Tumors per Rat	Rats with 3 or more Tumors
DMBA	79.0 (30/38)	2.8	47%
DMBA + 20% Bran	70.0 (28/40)	3.1	36%
DMBA + 0.4% IP_6	52.6 (20/38)	2.2	15%

Numbers in parentheses refer to the number of tumors per total number of animals. DMBA = 7,12-dimethylbenz[a] anthracene. Adapted from Vucenik, Yang, and Shamsuddin (1997).

substances, in this case the 20% bran diet. For cancer prevention, taking pure IP_6 thus may be a more sensible approach than having to gorge on enormous quantities of fiber. This was exactly what was said in an article in the *Washington Post* (March 14, 1989) which reported on my research published previously in the medical journal *Carcinogenesis*. "The American population may not have to gorge itself on fiber to prevent cancer after all," said the *Post* reporter, Larry Thompson.

Why is it more sensible to take pure IP_6 rather than bran? The explanations are simple. In the whole fiber or bran, or in cereals, IP_6 is bound to protein. For the IP_6 to be absorbed from the gut and transported in the bloodstream to the various organs and sites where cancer or disease has occurred or where it is likely to take hold, IP$_6$ must first be released from the protein complexes. There is an enzyme called phytase that is present in food and also found in the intestine. This enzyme can break down or degrade IP$_6$, making it inactive against cancer. The longer it takes IP$_6$ to be released from the whole fiber, the more time is available for the enzyme to degrade IP$_6$. So even though a high-fiber diet may contain high amounts of IP$_6$, you may never get the full benefit. Pure IP$_6$ is much better, since it will be absorbed before the enzyme has a chance to destroy it.

As regards any possible side effects, we checked the weight of all of the animals (that had been taking in the same amount of calories). Weights were similar in all groups and were not affected either by the addition of the bran to the diet, or IP$_6$ in the drinking water. Because of the concern that chronic administration of fiber or IP$_6$ might cause mineral deficiency (see above), we measured the blood serum levels of calcium, magnesium, zinc, and iron. The levels of these minerals were not significantly affected by fiber supplementation or with IP$_6$ treatment.

A similar study on breast cancer was done by Hirose and coworkers at Nagoya City University, Nagoya, Japan (1994). Again, rats were given the carcinogen DMBA with and without IP$_6$. Although this study used IP$_6$ added to the food, there was still a lower incidence of tumors, longer survival times, and fewer tumors per rat. The rats receiving the IP$_6$-rich diet also lived longer and with virtually no side effects. The IP$_6$ dietary supplement plan worked.

CHAPTER 4

IP$_6$: How Does It Protect Us?

It's in the Genes: Protecting Your DNA

Cell division is the basic means by which all living beings grow and reproduce. An organism that starts out as one cell will divide and there will be two "daughter" cells. A human fertilized egg begins to divide to form an embryo, which grows as cells divide further to become a fetus. An adult human must manufacture millions and millions of new cells continuously. Some tissues and organs continuously undergo cell division. For example, our skin cells are constantly replaced, as are cells that line the digestive tract. New red blood cells are needed continually, and organs such as the liver demand refurbishing. If cell division stops, such as happens with a large dose of ionizing radiation (as in nuclear bomb blast), death quickly happens.

Cell divisions are normally well regulated; the cell divides and the two new cells grow and develop. When there is abnormal, excessive, or unregulated cell division, however, a dangerous potential exists. This out-of-control cell division is the harbinger of cancer.

When cells divide, most will duplicate their contents (as mentioned in Chapter 3). The most important requirement here is for the genetic material, the DNA (deoxyribonucleic acid), to be faithfully replicated or copied. The DNA resides in the nucleus of the cell. The nucleus of the cell is separated from the rest of the cell by a surrounding membrane; it keeps the genetic material isolated and somewhat protected. After replication, the DNA will be distributed to each of the daughter cells. The daughter cells will then be genetically identical. For this to happen, new DNA must be made. DNA is composed of a chain of chemical building blocks containing what are called "bases." These bases are named adenine (A), guanine (G), cytosine (C), and thymine (T). The letters in parentheses are the symbols for the bases. These bases are strung together to form the DNA strand:

-A-G-C-T-G-A-C-T-, etc.

The arrangement of the bases is different for different species of living organisms. Two of these strands are wound together with the bases paired: A to G and C to T. When the DNA is ready to be copied, the strands unwind. New bases line up to match those on the original strand.

It is possible to tell when DNA synthesis is taking place by providing the cells with one such building block that is tagged with a radioactive substance. Measurement of how much of the tagged bases are used allows us to get an idea about the rate of DNA synthesis. Thymidine (a combination of the base thymine + the sugar, ribose) is used by cells exclusively for DNA synthesis. We did experiments in my laboratory with radioactively labeled thymidine (^{3}H-thymidine). It was incorporated into the DNA. When we measured how much labeled thymidine was taken up, we saw a reduction in DNA synthesis that was brought about by IP_6. We also saw a decrease in the process of actual division of the genetic material and the cell nucleus (mitosis). It is reasonable to conclude from this and from other studies that I will discuss later that IP_6 is effective in controlling cell division.

Antioxidant Protection: Iron Is Out

In addition to functions that have already been discussed, IP_6 is also an antioxidant and many of its beneficial actions can be attributed to this property. So what is an antioxidant and why is it "anti-"?

For humans and most other organisms, oxygen is essential for life. In the human body, however, the amounts and activity of oxygen need to be regulated. Cells and components within the cell (the intracellular components) may be injured if there is too much oxygen (O_2 is the symbol for the oxygen molecule with the number two indicating that there are two oxygen atoms bonded together). When atoms interact with one another, chemical reactions take place that can generate entities called "free radicals." Atoms have electrically charged particles called electrons circling the nucleus or center of the atom. An atom is in its "most favorite" energy state when its electrons are paired. The oxygen molecule (O_2) has an equal number of shared electrons and is thus "content." When one electron is pulled away from the molecule, however, the atom with its unpaired electron is "discontented." It actively seeks another electron to pair with and will take it from another atom or molecule. Such a reactive, electron-seeking atom or molecule is called a free radical. Singlet oxygen (written $O_2^{\bullet-}$, oxygen with one electron), is a high-energy and highly reactive form of oxygen molecule. The dot ($\bullet$) indicates the unpaired electron, resulting in a net negative charge as indicated by the negative sign. Singlet oxygen is also called activated oxygen or reactive oxygen species. There are other free radicals besides $O_2^{\bullet-}$, such as hydrogen peroxide (H_2O_2 with unpaired 2 electrons) and hydroxyl radical ($\bullet OH$ with three unpaired electrons). Together these reactive species form the group called superoxides. These superoxides can damage the DNA, proteins, and other molecules in the cells by oxidizing them. The chemical reaction that produces this damage is called an oxidation reaction. The free radicals produced are called oxidants. Antioxidants, as the name implies, are "anti-" the oxidants, hence the name *antioxidants*. The antioxidants stop the oxidants by giving them the electron they need, thus preventing any possible damage down the road. You have heard of the antioxidants such as ascorbate (vitamin C), the vitamin E family (tocopherols), and carotenoids (such as beta-carotene and lycopene, etc.). IP$_6$ is also an antioxidant, and a strong one at that.

Free radicals are not always bad; their properties can be used for good causes. They are produced by neutrophils, the immune system cells that engulf bacteria and other invaders when they venture into our body. These cells use the superoxides and other free radicals for the actual killing of bacteria. They keep these reactive species stored in tiny "bags" within the cell. Thus protected, the free radicals will not harm other structures in the cell and also will not be inactivated by antioxidants. They are waiting like bombs to be dropped on the enemy. But free radicals are like a double-edged sword—they can be protective, but an excessive or unusual accumulation of free radicals can be equally damaging to the host; that is, *us.* As if our internal sources for free radicals are not enough, they can be generated from external sources as well. Cigarette smoke, UV radiation from the sun, excessive oxygen therapy, the radiation used for cancer therapy, drugs, etc., are all potent generating sources. Even our daily normal diets can give us a dose of free radicals when foods are metabolized.

The damage, or oxidative damage, caused by free radicals can harm the DNA. Such harm can cause mutations in the genetic material, leading to a host of diseases, from cancer to cataracts. Even aging, in part, is a result of the damage caused by free radicals. In the extreme situation, the unrepaired DNA damage may prevent the cell from replicating or copying its own DNA. That may not be of much consequence if the cells in question do not have to divide. But if the cells must divide, the inability to replicate the DNA results in the death of the cell. Normally, oxidative damage in the DNA strand is cut out (excised) and repaired by enzymes in the body. However, if oxidative damages and mutations build up in the DNA over a length of time, as they tend to, this can pose serious problems, such as cancer and other diseases associated with aging. Dr. Bruce Ames and his colleagues (1993) have done much research on free radicals and aging. They and many other researchers have learned that when cells and their DNA are not protected by antioxidants, these diseases and aging are accelerated.

How does IP$_6$ perform as an antioxidant? All cells contain numerous small structures that are the "energy factories" in each cell (the mitochondria). In the mitochondria, using compounds that originally came from the diet and have been broken down for fuel, a series of chemical reactions takes place. These reactions ultimately produce the energy that keeps us alive. This process of changing fuel into energy is called respiration (not the same as the term used for breathing). Cells respire by transferring electrons from one molecule to another in the mitochondria, and the mineral iron is essential for this reaction to happen. Cells get this iron from the blood plasma. As a by-product of this reaction, free radicals are produced. Some are necessary for the reaction but others are made in excess with the potential for creating havoc. Hydrogen peroxide (H_2O_2) is formed during respiration and reacts with iron in a process called the Fenton reaction to produce reactive and damaging hydroxyl radicals ($\bullet OH$).

IP$_6$ removes excess iron at the reaction site by binding with it, thus inhibiting $\bullet OH$ generation from the Fenton reaction. This stops a subsequently harmful reaction called lipid peroxidation—or damage caused to the lipids (or fats) that are a part of the cell membranes. It happens when free radicals attack the membrane lipid molecules. Embedded in the cell membrane are molecules formed from fatty acids and phosphates—such as phosphatidyl inositol biphosphate (PIP_2)—called phospholipids. In the membrane the combination of the two is called phosphatidyl inositol. The DNA is also protected from free radical damage. By binding up (chelating) iron, IP_6 has the unique ability to remove O_2 without allowing the formation of oxygen free radicals.

In an experiment conducted by my colleagues at the University of Maryland School of Medicine, Drs. Mary J. Hinzman and Peter L. Gutierrez, using a technique called electron spin resonance spectroscopy, it was demonstrated that IP_6 reduces free radical formation. With the addition of IP_6, the free radical level was reduced by more than 2½ times. IP_6 reduced the active oxygen species-mediated cancer formation and cell injury by its antioxidative function. In Chapter 6, I will provide direct evidence as to how IP_6 can stop the damaging consequences of free radicals by using a common example of asbestos-induced lung destruction.

In the plant kingdom IP_6 also functions as an antioxidant, protecting and preserving the seeds, which may remain viable (alive and able to grow) for a long time. The arrangement of the phosphates in the IP_6 molecule uniquely provides a specific interaction with iron (as mentioned above) to completely inhibit its ability to help produce hydroxyl free radicals. Protection against cancer, cardiovascular diseases, cataracts and a multitude of other applications of IP_6 are the result of this beneficial antioxidant function.

CHAPTER 5

IP$_6$: Action Against Cancer

The Cancer Problem

Cancer is a major public health problem worldwide, with 6.6 million people dying yearly. In the United States alone, it is estimated that 560,000 people die of cancer every year, and nearly 1.4 million new cases are diagnosed annually. Over 25 years ago President Richard M. Nixon declared "War on Cancer." Since then the government and private sector have spent enormous amounts of money to learn what we now know about the biology of the disease. Despite the continued optimism, however, we haven't made much gain in the battlefield, let alone win the war. But from time to time, we have had our share of excitement. Battlefield strategies were, and continue to be, devised by the generals: in this case, our leaders in cancer research. The decision makers at the National Cancer Institute, the American Cancer Society, and other like organizations choose the targets and support the scientific community in its efforts to develop "silver bullets" or "guided missiles" to attack the cancer cells.

Scientists have responded well to the strategy advanced; for they find within it funding to do their research. New therapies such as the use of monoclonal antibodies to target cancer cells and immune system—boosting interleukin and interferon to inhibit cancer spread were developed. These therapies and the scientists who developed them, prompted national recognition and much discussion in the popular media. Yet the menace of cancer continues. Innovative research that deviates from the mainstream development of new cancer drugs and radiation therapies is not as likely to be appreciated or even funded. My research, like that of many independent scientists who do not follow the status quo however, has also brought with it new therapies and new hope for success in our war against cancer. Dr. Arthur Kornberg, an eminent molecular biologist, in a recent editorial in *Science* (December 12, 1997) has put it this way: "A common *illusion* [italics mine] is that strategic objectives are necessary to discover the cure for cancer and AIDS and that groups of sufficient size need to be mobilized for wars and crusades against these enemies. *Nothing could be more misguided* [italics mine]. In the history of triumphs in biomedical research such wars and crusades have invariably failed because they lacked the necessary weapons— the essential knowledge of basic life processes. Instead, some of the major advances—X-rays, penicillin, polio vaccine, and genetic engineering—have come from the efforts of individual scientists to understand Nature. . . ."

So what have I discovered about IP₆ and cancer?

My research results with animals and, most importantly, on human cancer cells, are exciting. Together with
what we already know about the benefits and safety
of inositol in humans, the combination of IP$_6$ and
inositol can give cancer a one, two punch! A wise
man once said, "What you find on the road you travel
to reach your goal is often just as important as the
goal itself." Let's go down that road.

Cancer Prevention

Until I began my research, no one had asked the
question, "What role does IP$_6$ play in the prevention
of cancer?" In response, I had to devise an experiment that would give me some answers to build on.
Usually in experiments on nutrition and cancer, the
nutrient (IP$_6$ in this case) would be added to the food.
My experience in pharmacology, however, indicated
that adding IP$_6$ in its pure form to the drinking water
of the experimental animals would allow for better
absorption. Since rats cannot be given a pure supplement as a tablet or capsule, and I did not want other
food substances to interfere with the IP$_6$, it was put
in water. This would be equivalent to a human taking
an oral supplement with water, between meals. My
first thought was also a humane one: I would try it
myself before I gave the IP$_6$ solution to the rats. It
tasted just fine. Since inositol has the chemical structure of a sugar, it is slightly sweet. The rats would
probably like it!

Initially I had to find the most drinkable IP$_6$ solution for the rats. I found that they would drink it
only at a concentration of 5% or less. The best dose
was somewhat less, up to 2% solution, which enabled

them to drink their normal, daily amount of water. Compared to a human of 150 pounds, this solution would be equal to about 1 to 2 grams (1000 to 2000 milligrams) of IP$_6$ taken orally. To determine the effectiveness of IP$_6$ in different species and against tumors produced by different carcinogens, we used different animals (rats and mice) and different chemicals (1,2-dimethylhydrazine and azoxymethane) that cause colon cancer.

We began by giving IP$_6$ to the rats 2 weeks before starting carcinogen administration. This was during the preinitiation phase in order to give the treatment time to start working. We gave the rats 1% IP$_6$, an amount equal to 500 milligrams to 1000 milligrams oral dose in a 150-pound human. (See Chapter 3 for an explanation of the phases of cancer progression.) We also wanted to see if treatment with IP$_6$ would cancel out the carcinogenic action. Six months later, the average number of tumors in the control rats (those not given IP$_6$) was 4.6 per animal, while for the IP$_6$-treated animals the tumor number was 3.0. Also, the tumors were approximately two-thirds smaller in the animals receiving the IP$_6$. Early in the experiment I also saw another effect of IP$_6$. In the IP$_6$-treated animals who had tumors, the rate of cell division in the nontumorous colon cells was similar to that of the normal control animals. In other words, the carcinogen-induced increase in cell division was normalized, indicating a regulatory function of IP$_6$. Most interestingly, the cell division rate of the animals receiving IP$_6$ treatment without the carcinogen was normal. This suggests that IP$_6$ simply brings down the elevated rate of cell division during cancer formation, but does not affect the normal rate of cell division in otherwise healthy animals. Here indeed was a statistically significant result—the type of result accepted by all expert researchers! The details of these experiments are found in my research publications in 1988, 1989, and 1990 (see the Bibliography). Since the maximal dose of carcinogen was used in this initial experiment, with the animals developing tumors, there was significant inhibition of tumor size.

When I saw these results, that the tumor size in IP$_6$-treated animals was smaller, I knew that IP$_6$ might be effective even after cancer had already taken hold (during the postinitiation phase). Consequently, IP$_6$ was given to rats as early as 2 weeks after, or as late as 5 months following, carcinogen administration. My coworkers and I showed that the inhibition of colon cancer was also seen even when the carcinogen was given 2 weeks or 5 months before IP$_6$ treatment. It is also important to note that since we started the IP$_6$ treatment later, I decided to give a higher dose (2%) than what was given in the previous experiment (i.e. 1%).

Eight months after 4 doses of the carcinogen azoxymethane was given, only 10% of the animals on IP$_6$ developed colon cancer, compared to 43% in the group not receiving IP$_6$. Compounds that contain the prefix "azo-" are highly reactive with other molecules, such as those in human or animal tissue. Azo dyes, for example (those that are yellow), are very damaging to cells. Animals showed significantly lower tumor number and tumor size even when given IP$_6$ up to 5 months after cancer initiation, a time when most of the animals are expected to have cancers. These findings pointed toward the possible therapeutic use of IP$_6$ for existing cancer.

Table 4 shows the data on the tumor frequency and mitotic rates (an indication of cell division), as lowered by IP_6.

Table 4.
Colon Cancer Inhibition After 5 Months

Treatments	No. of Tumors per Rat	Mitotic Rate, %
AOM only	7.1	2.3
AOM + IP_6	5.2	1.0

AOM = the carcinogen, azoxymethane.

We then wanted to see whether there was a dose-dependent reduction in large intestine cancer with IP_6—whether giving more IP_6 worked even better. My colleague, Asad Ullah, and I (1990) tested doses as low as 0.1% and 1% IP_6 (equivalent to oral doses of 100 milligrams and 1000 milligrams in a 150-pound human). We showed that the prevalence of tumors decreases with increasing IP_6 dosage. Figure 3 shows the results of the dose-dependence study. The rats were started on IP_6 2 weeks before being injected with 6 doses of the carcinogen azoxymethane (AOM). Note here a dose-related decrease in tumor prevalence of 52.2% with 1.0% IP_6 at the end of the experiment at 44 weeks.

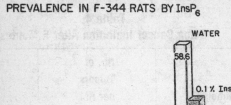

Figure 3.
Dose-dependent effect

The figure shows that the highest tumor incidence in rats given the carcinogen azoxymethane (AOM) was for rats given water without IP₆ (the control animals). Rats given 0.1% IP₆ had a lower incidence of cancer, while rats receiving 1% IP₆ (equivalent to between 1 to 2 grams in oral form for a human) resulted in the lowest incidence of cancer. IP₆ was given to rats at week 6 of the experiment, 2 weeks before AOM was given. AOM was given from week 8 to week 14. At 44 weeks, the tumor incidence in the rats was determined. LIC = Large Intestinal Cancer; InsP₆ is another abbreviation for inositol hexaphosphate (IP₆); Na-InsP₆ is the sodium (Na) salt of IP₆, the form of it found in solution.

Since IP_6 undergoes dephosphorylation to IP_{1-5} (see Chapter 3), and IP_3 is important as a cellular messenger, my theory was that IP_6 could enter into the inositol phosphate pool inside the cell. Inside the cell it would be converted to IP_3 and cause tumor suppression through the action of lower (number) inositol phosphates. I had also hypothesized, in 1988, that the addition of inositol, an innocuous natural carbohydrate from which IP_6 is formed, could enhance the anticancer function of IP_6. Because inositol phosphates are ubiquitous (found everywhere) and are involved in the function of most mammalian cell systems, I believed that the anticancer action of inositol phosphates would be observed in different cells and organs.

By the end of 1987, I had demonstrated the following:

- IP_6 prevented colon cancer in two different species of animals (rats and mice).
- Inositol is also cancer inhibitory, although by itself it is much less efficient than IP_6.
- IP_6 + inositol are better than either one of them alone (a synergistic combination).
- IP_6 + inositol enhanced host resistance (immunity) by stimulating the activity of natural killer (NK) cells, the immune system cells that fight cancer.
- IP_6 is effective against a *human* cancer cell line (K-562 human erythroleukemia).

I then wished to determine whether the antitumor action of IP_6 involved the less phosphorylated forms of inositol which are important in cell division. I also wanted to see whether the addition of inositol would enhance the antiproliferative and thus the anticancer action of IP$_6$.

In support of my belief that the antitumor action of IP$_6$ involves lower IPs, my coworkers and I conducted a further experiment. We treated K-562 human erythroleukemia cells with IP$_6$. We chose these human leukemia cells because we knew that these cells would make hemoglobin (as red blood cells do) if the IP$_6$ acted to normalize the cells. We did find that hemoglobin levels increased in the cells treated with IP$_6$, but not in untreated K-562 cells. This meant that the cells were reverting to a more normal or mature type. The number of cells decreased with IP$_6$ treatment, indicating a reduced ability of the cells to multiply at an abnormal rate.

In addition to showing that IP$_6$ gets into the K-562 cells, we also found that there is a significant (41%) increase in IP$_3$ inside the cell. We know that IP$_6$ is converted to these lower forms in the cell. This experiment and others point to the rapid conversion of IP$_6$ to inositol and IP$_{1.5}$. It is clear then that giving IP$_6$ changes the amounts of the different inositol phosphates inside the cells. We also know that these changes inside the cell relate to stopping cell division. Now the level of calcium inside a cell affects the growth rate of that cell. For its part, IP$_6$ causes an increase of calcium inside the cell. While many studies show that an increase in calcium concentration may result in cell division, our data shows the opposite: a *decrease* in cell division. Resolution of this dilemma may depend on the amounts of IP$_3$ present in the cell. Usually, IP$_3$ increases cell division. We think, however, with higher levels of inositol and IP$_6$

given, that IP_3 could be inhibited and so is cell division, and the risk of cancer, decreased. Recently my associates Dr. Katharine E. Cole and Mary Smith (1997) have demonstrated that, within 10 seconds after adding IP_6 to human colon tumor cells, there is a rapid three- to four-fold rise in calcium in the cell. This fast increase in calcium strongly suggests that IP_6 is acting on a receptor in the cell. In this case, evidence points to IP_6 having an action that may block a receptor for a growth. With this receptor blocked, the cancer cell cannot grow and multiply.

The inference here was found correct! Inositol enhanced the ability of IP_6 to inhibit cell division as well as its antitumor effect *in vivo* (in the living body). A significantly greater suppression of both cell proliferation and colorectal cancer was also noted when inositol was added to IP_6. This same enhancement effect was seen in the mammary cancer and metastatic tumor experiments by my colleague Dr. Ivana Vucenik (1992, 1993). A long-standing collaborator, Dr. Ivana Vucenik worked tirelessly, and with very little financial support, to conclude her experiments. Dr. Kosaku Sakamoto, a surgeon from Gunma University, Japan, also worked tirelessly in my laboratory, compelled by the therapeutic possibilities he saw in the experiments.

Were other IP_6 researchers getting the same results? I was pleased to learn that they were. Dr. Raxit Jariwalla at the Linus Pauling Institute in Palo Alto, California, had confirmed my observations of the anticancer action of IP_6. Dr. Theresa Pretlow, from Case Western Reserve University in Cleveland, Ohio, also came to the same statistically significant conclusions as I had. As she wrote:

The incidence of tumors in F344 rats treated with AOM without phytate was 83% (10/12) compared to 25% (3/12) in rats treated with AOM plus phytate ...

—T. P. Pretlow et al. (1992)

The Pretlow group also reported their results at the Third Annual Conference on Nutrition and Cancer by the American Institute for Cancer Research, October 29-30, 1992, in Mclean, Virginia. They said that not only was IP$_6$ an effective inhibitor of colon cancer, but that it was also more effective when compared to other candidate chemopreventive agents, such as selenium. "Colon Carcinogenesis Is Inhibited *More Effectively by Phytate* [italics mine] than by Selenium in F344 Rats Given 30 mg/kg Azoxymethane," reads the title of the article published in *Advances in Experimental Medicine and Biology* in 1994.

There is another compelling indication of the importance of IP$_6$. Its antitumor (antineoplastic) action may not be restricted to the colon. This has been demonstrated by us and others (see Chapter 6, Table 5, and Chapter 10, Table 9). In some of these experiments, of course, the method of giving IP$_6$ varied. When given in the form of bran (as phytate), it was not as biologically active as when given in pure form as IP$_6$ or as IP$_6$ + inositol. Because of its ability to form complexes with proteins, preventing its action, addition of IP$_6$ to food may explain the slight difference in results obtained by different investigators.

How Does IP$_6$ Work?

The exact mechanism(s) through which IP$_6$ exerts its antitumor effects are not yet known. We must remember that scientists in the field of nutrition and agriculture were previously not looking at IP_6 for its benefits. Instead, they were preoccupied with the possible "toxicity" of IP_6 based on old and inadequate information about the mineral-chelating ability of phytate. As we discussed in Chapter 2 and will discuss further in Chapter 8, this ability of phytate nonetheless is not a problem and can often be beneficial in the case of iron. There was also a lack of interactive research between nutrition scientists, cell biologists and biochemists. In fact, no one seemed able to grasp the whole picture; they were looking elsewhere. Others had ignored IP_6 altogether (as discussed by F. S. Menniti and colleagues in 1993). It was even thought that IP_6 could not be absorbed by organisms, much less that it might act in the cell. Preliminary work by Nahapetian and Young (1980) showing evidence of its absorption was ignored, as were the facts that it was present in the cell and that there were various mechanisms to transport IP_6 molecules across cell membranes and into the cells!

Since cancer is a major public health issue, the dramatic anticancer effect of IP_6 prompts us to understand its mechanism of action. As a first step in this quest, studies in my laboratory have demonstrated that, contrary to popular misconception, IP_6 is very quickly absorbed from the stomach and upper small intestine of rats and distributed to various organs as early as 1 hour following administration (Sakamoto, Vucenik, and Shamsuddin, 1993). Using radioactive tracers we note that inositol and all the forms of inositol + phosphate (IP_{1-6}) can be found in the stomach lining. In the blood plasma and urine we see inositol and IP_1. Finding this molecule with fewer phosphate groups attached indicates that the body rapidly metabolizes the compound. The presence of IP$_6$ in the stomach lining also suggests that it is transported intact to the inside of the cell wherein it is rapidly dephosphorylated.

In this regard, it is unlikely that IP$_6$ is dephosphorylated outside the cell and then absorbed as inositol and IP$_{1-5}$ which then combines to make IP$_6$ inside the cell. Cutting off the phosphate groups requires the action of an enzyme, mucosal phytase. There is no mucosal phytase activity in the stomach—so this enzyme is not present to do the job of cutting up the molecule. In our experiments, we were careful to fast the animals for 2 hours to avoid action of any phytase enzyme that could be taken in with food. And although we did not demonstrate conclusively that intact IP$_6$ is transported inside the cell, the evidence is in favor of such an event.

Studies of the absorption of IP$_6$ by malignant cells *in vitro* also demonstrate that the cells almost instantaneously begin to accumulate IP$_6$, the rate of accumulation varying for the different types of cells (Vucenik and Shamsuddin, 1994). For instance, the uptake of IP$_6$ by the mouse YAC-1 lymphoma cell line leveled off as early as 10 minutes after cells were exposed. The ability and the rate at which the cells metabolized IP$_6$ also varied; YAC-1 and human K-562 cells contained only the lower inositol phosphates, whereas HT-29 human colon carcinoma cells had inositol and IP$_{1-6}$. Interestingly, the growth rate of these cells are also different. The human HT-29 colon cancer cells (with inositol + IP$_{1-6}$) grew the slowest while the other cancer cell lines grew the fastest.

When IP$_6$ forms complexes with various proteins and other molecules, its absorption and metabolic activation slows, especially when IP$_6$ is taken in only as part of the diet—along with all other food components. Giving it in pure form by mouth, however, is likely to be more effective. Indeed, comparison of various studies lends support to this idea. For instance, we saw a similar level of tumor inhibition with a small amount of IP_6 given every other day (Vucenik et al., 1992) as compared to other researchers who gave a larger amount of IP_6 mixed in the diet (Jariwalla et al., 1988). Likewise, Hirose and colleagues (1991) did not see significant inhibition of colon tumors by dietary IP_6 although they did see a slight inhibition of liver and pancreatic tumor development.

Finally, IP_6 can combat cancer by boosting the activity of natural killer (NK) cells. These are immune system cells (also called lymphocytes) that can kill tumor cells as well as help in the body's fight against a variety of chronic infectious diseases. The effect of IP_6 in boosting the NK cell activity will be discussed in detail in Chapter 6. Since NK cells play an important role in host defense against tumors (neoplasia), it is quite likely that IP_6 exerts its antineoplastic action by increasing its ability to kill cancer cells (NK-cell cytotoxicity).

For a more detailed discussion on other possible mechanisms of action of IP_6, see Chapter 6, which describes the work of Huang and colleagues (1997), and Shamsuddin and colleagues (1997).

Cancer Therapy and IP$_6$

Treating Cancer Cells

Our experiments were clear and persuasive: colorectal cancer was inhibited when IP$_6$ treatment was
begun as late as 5 months following initiation. We
thus realized something more: IP$_6$ could work in the
treatment of *existing* cancers. Perhaps IP$_6$ was not
restricted just to the prevention of tumor development. The fact the IP$_6$ normalizes cell division rate
provided additional impetus for us—we would plan
new experiments.

In fully developed cancers as well as in early stage
cancer, cell numbers increase. Thus, we planned laboratory tests to determine the therapeutic properties
of IP$_6$ in mice that already had tumors. These tumors
resulted from injection under the skin with cancerous
mouse fibrosarcoma (FSA-1) cells. A fibrosarcoma is
a cancerous tumor made of fibrous connective tissue,
and which tends to invade nearby tissues and also

spread (metastasize) by tumor cells carried in the bloodstream. Intravenous injection of the FSA-1 cells, for instance, caused the tumor to spread to the lung. Treatment of the mice with injections of IP$_6$ every other day, however, resulted in both a significant inhibition of tumor size and improvement of survival time over the mice that did not receive IP$_6$. The injection contained 0.25% IP$_6$, equivalent to an oral dose of about 125–250 milligrams in a 150-pound person. When these mice with tumors were treated with IP$_6$ there was a significant reduction in the number of tumors that had spread to the lung (metastatic lung colonies) as we reported in the journal, *Cancer Letters* (Vucenik et al., 1992). In summary, the data from this experiment shows that IP$_6$ not only prevents cancer, but exerts an anticancer effect against established cancer and also against advanced cancer that has spread to another location in the body. The experiment showed that continuous treatment with IP$_6$ is critical for obtaining the best antitumor effect. In preparation for future clinical trials in humans, we also studied the safety of IP$_6$ administration and found it happily as nontoxic in long-term supplementation.

With an experiment similar to ours, but in rats, Jariwalla and his colleagues (1988) have also reported parallel results. They gave a much higher dose of IP$_6$, however, since it was added to the diet. As I mentioned earlier, IP$_6$ can interact with proteins in the diet and become less available. Giving it in a pure form allows maximum absorption and effect. Dr. Jariwalla also found no evidence of toxicity and the study results also indicated that IP$_6$ may have a beneficial effect in lowering cholesterol and triglycerides buildup.

IP$_6$ also has an effect on cancer cell lines. These

are populations of cancer cells that were taken from tumors and maintained (or cultured) in the laboratory. *In vitro* studies of both human and rodent cancer cell lines in my laboratory show that IP$_6$ reduces cell proliferation rate in all of the cell lines tested; the cells do not keep multiplying. Interestingly, unlike most other anticancer agents, with IP$_6$ the cells do not show an overwhelming evidence of cytotoxicity; that is, the cells are not dying from having too much IP$_6$ around. Instead, the growth of the cancerous (malignant) cells slows. The cells become mature and then they die. But let us pause for a moment to understand why it is important for a cancer cell to mature.

Many cancer cells resemble immature cells such as those seen in a fetus. These cells have not yet developed into a specialized cell, such as a skin cell or a heart cell. These immature cells have the potential to become any one of a number of different cell types. An immature cancer cell is also more aggressive—it divides and multiplies faster. More mature cancer cells, meaning they look more like cells that have already specialized or differentiated (such as liver cells, lung cells, skin cells, etc.), on the other hand, are usually less aggressive. A cell that has a "normal phenotype" looks like what it was intended to be; that is, a skin cell, a kidney cell, or other type of cell. The word *phenotype* refers to the appearance of the cell.

The reduced cell growth and enhanced maturation, or differentiation, of cancer cells to the point of reversion back to normal phenotype is seen in different cell lines. For instance, K-562 human erythroleukemia cells are relatively small compared to their normal counterpart, the erythrocytes (red blood cells); and they have no hemoglobin (the molecule that carries iron in a red blood cell). With IP$_6$ treatment, a striking growth inhibition of the erythroleukemia cells was achieved. In addition, few of these cells remained alive 48 hours after the start of treatment. At lower concentrations of IP$_6$, the effect was somewhat different, with cells staying alive for a longer period of time. Be that as it may, their numbers were reduced, they grew in size, and accumulated hemoglobin, becoming more like mature cells, in this case red blood cells (Shamsuddin and colleagues, 1992). The study also found that after 3 months of continuous treatment with IP$_6$, there was a 21% reduction of cell population. Even with noncontinuous treatment (every third or fourth day), the results were similar.

That IP$_6$ (with or without inositol) causes the cancer cells to behave normally is similar to a social situation. Let's say the cancer cells are our youths gone angry, forming a gang (the cancer) and eating up the society by their destructive behavior. Some in our society would like to give them the death sentence . . . just like we would like to kill the cancer cells. But it may not be possible to kill all the cancer cells, or doing so may cause severe toxic effects in the body of the person treated. An alternative plan, in the case of society's misfits described above, is to educate and rehabilitate them and bring them back into civilized society, so that they, too, become productive members.

IP$_6$ does exactly that—it causes the cancer cells to mature and to behave like normal cells. Now, in the research laboratory we can look under the microscope and say that the tumor cells have been tamed. But how do we know that IP$_6$ treatment can bring our cells back to normal in a living, walking, talking, human being?

This is how: Many cancer cells, including those of the colon, breast, prostate, lungs, pancreas, to name a few, express a marker that is otherwise not expressed by normal healthy cells or in normal people. This marker is a simple sugar, made of 2 units of galactose ß-D-galactose-[1 → 3]-N-acetyl-galactos-amine. Now that's too long and difficult a name; so we shall call it Gal-GalNAc for short. While cells of normal people do not express Gal-GalNAc, the mucous sample from the colon of a person harboring a cancer expresses it, as I discuss in my article in *Anticancer Research* (1995). I had invented a test (a very simple one) that detects Gal-GalNAc, and hence colon cancer. It tests the rectal mucus for this marker with 80-100% sensitivity and specificity; in other words, the test can detect low amounts of the marker and specifically that marker alone. The test is currently used extensively in China. For more details, see Zhou and colleagues (1991).

Let's say a patient with cancer of the colon with cells expressing the marker Gal-GalNAc in the rectal mucus has had the cancer surgically removed. Patients who have undergone such surgery also have a much higher risk of getting a second cancer in the same place—in this instance, the colon—later on. To prevent the possibility of any surprise here, of a second cancer appearing unmonitored, he or she could be periodically tested for Gal-GalNAc. Since this person was previously positive for Gal-GalNAc, a negative test at a later time would indicate that he or she is free of cancer cells in the colon or any risk of it. If IP$_6$ would indeed reduce the risk and prevent cancer formation, wouldn't it be nice if it could simultaneously suppress Gal-GalNAc expression? If it did, we could monitor the effect.

That's not just wishful thinking. To test that possibility we used a HT-29 human colon cancer cell line. In the summer of 1992, a second-year medical student, Giridhar Venkatraman, came to me to do a research project. After I familiarized him with the two projects—IP_6 and the test for Gal-GalNAc—he simply said that he wanted to work on both! His enthusiasm as much as his choice impressed me—and I began to think.

Gal-GalNAc is expressed by HT-29 (the marker is within the mucus of these cells). Wouldn't it be great if IP_6 did suppress Gal-GalNAc in these cells? Dr. Kosaku Sakamoto, a surgeon from Gunma University, Japan, was working in my laboratory at that time. Dr. Sakamoto had left his successful practice to work in my lab for 2 years without salary, simply because he believed in the research. During that summer we found that, as a result of IP_6 treatment, along with an inhibition of cell proliferation, the expression of the tumor marker Gal-GalNAc by these cells was also markedly suppressed. In most cells no expression whatsoever could be seen even though the cells produced the mucus (Sakamoto and colleagues, 1993). Producing mucus indicates that the cells are mature. Thus, while IP_6 suppresses the malignant or cancerous cell form, it still allows normal function—the production of mucus. IP_6 lets the human colon cancer cells mature so that they structurally and behaviorally resemble normal cells. Again, our results showed that IP_6 was safe.

Dr. Guang-Yu Yang from the China Medical University in Shenyang later joined my laboratory. He, too, confirmed that IP_6 caused cancer cells to normalize and not express tumor markers (Yang and Shamsuddin, 1995). Thus, in the scenario we have just discussed, testing for Gal-GalNAc could be used to determine how well IP$_6$ was working against cancer. In addition, the test could be used to check on the effectiveness of other anticancer agents that cause cells to mature or differentiate.

Which Cancers Could Be Treated by IP$_6$?

There is a commonly used measure to depict the efficacy of a drug or other substance. It is called the Inhibitory Concentration (IC) and comes into play when there is a 50% inhibition of cell number—the IC$_{50}$. The doses or the concentration required to achieve IC$_{50}$ vary for the different types of cells or cell lines. While cells of the blood cell forming (hematopoietic) line (e.g. K-562 human erythroleukemia, YAC-1 mouse lymphoma, or HL-60 human leukemia) are highly sensitive to IP$_6$, those of the skin and body cavity lining (epithelial) and connective tissue, blood vessel, and lymph tissue (mesenchymal) lines appear to require higher concentrations of IP$_6$. Using cancerous connective tissue cells (BALB/c mouse 3T3 fibroblasts) and testing for cell toxicity, Babich and colleagues (1993) compared the effects of several nutrients with cancer preventive effects. They found a moderate cell toxicity with IP$_6$; it was not killing the cells. This modest result is not surprising since extensive experiments with human cancer cell lines *in vitro* in my laboratory show little cytotoxicity as well. Whether they are cancerous or healthy, IP$_6$ doesn't kill cells. Cancer drugs, on the other hand, do kill cells without discrimination—both cancer and normal cells. IP_6 stops cancer cells from growing uncontrollably and normalizes them.

Furthermore, while inositol alone works modestly against cancer *in vivo* (Shamsuddin and Ullah, 1989; Estensen and Wattenberg, 1993; Vucenik et al., 1993), when added to IP_6 there is a synergistic effect. In other words, IP_6 given together with inositol works much better against cancer cells than either nutrient alone. (See Chapter 10 for more details.)

The results of the animal experiments showing how well IP_6 works against various cancers are given in Chapter 10. In Table 5, there is a summary of the cancer cell lines that have been tested *in vitro*, and found to be inhibited significantly by IP_6. Based on our extensive testing, it is highly likely that these cancers would be inhibited by IP_6 *in vivo*, in the living organism, as well.

The study by Huang and colleagues provide evidence for the mechanism of IP_6—what it is doing on a biochemical level to prevent or stop cancer. As mentioned earlier, IP_6 and its family of inositol phosphates are involved in a system of messenger cells. This system, also called a signal transduction pathway, can be activated by tumor promoters. It works like this: The tumor promoter activates protein 1 (AP-1), a critical component of tumor growth, by way of an enzyme: phosphatidyl inositol-3 (PI-3 kinase). IP_6, however, was found to have a structure very similar to a potent inhibitor of the enzyme (PI-3 kinase). IP_6, thus, works against, or inhibits, the tumor by blocking the action of the enzyme. And while cancer drugs could be developed to block PI-3 kinase, these same cancer drugs are inherently toxic. Not so with IP_6, significantly as well, the results of this study also showed that IP_6 may directly target PI-3 kinase.

Table 5.
Proven Effectiveness of IP$_6$ Against Different Cancer Cell Lines

Tissue or Organ Type	Cancer Cell Line
Brain tumor	SR.B10A[1]
Breast cancer	MCF-7[2]
	MDA-MB-231[2]
	MDA-MB-435[3]
Colon carcinoma	HT-29[4]
Erythroleukemia	K-562[5]
Fibroblast, immortalized	BALBc-3T3[6]
Liver carcinoma	Hep G2[7]
Lung carcinoma	HTB-119[3]
	RTE[8]
Mouse lymphoma	YAC-1[3]
Myeloid leukemia	HL-60[3]
Prostate carcinoma	PC-3[9]
Skeletal muscle sarcoma	RD[10]
Skin carcinoma	JB6[11]

1. Kosaku Sakamoto, Gunma University, Japan [unpublished].
2. Shamsuddin et al., 1996. 3. Work in my laboratory [unpublished].
4. Sakamoto et al., 1993, and Yang and Shamsuddin, 1995. 5. Shamsuddin et al., 1992. 6. Babich et al., 1993. 7. Tantivejkul et al., 1998. 8. Arnold et al., 1995. 9. Shamsuddin and Yang, 1995. 10. Vucenik et al., 1997b. 11. Huang et al., 1997.

Certainly, such results and others seen with IP$_6$ are most provocative—they challenge our current convictions and offer fresh possibilities for nontoxic, anticancer therapy. For instance, hormones, particularly estrogen, are considered to be of key importance in the formation and treatment of breast cancer.

Some breast cancers will respond to hormones by growing. In order to respond to a hormone, the tumor must have a receptor for the hormone—sort of docking station. As such, breast cancers are tested for the presence or absence of estrogen or progesterone receptors (ER or PR). MCF-7 breast cancer cells, for example, are estrogen receptor positive (meaning estrogen will bind to these receptors), whereas MDAMB-231 breast cancer cells are negative. Yet IP$_6$ is just as effective in inhibiting *both* of these cell lines. Conventionally, a breast tumor that is estrogen-positive must be treated differently from one that is not. In a similar light, PC-3 cells from prostate carcinoma are testosterone dependent (meaning they depend on testosterone for development). Like breast cancer, prostate cancer also has been treated by removing the hormone source; for example, by removing the testes in an operation called an orchiectomy, or by using chemicals to get rid of male hormones; but IP$_6$ causes a striking inhibition of these cells as well.

Clearly, IP$_6$ functions here by avoiding the hormone receptors, thereby making it effective for virtually any cell line. These actions of IP$_6$ have been observed during anticancer studies done by various other investigators. Jariwalla and colleagues, however, put it this way:

> Phytate [the salt of IP$_6$] addition highly significantly lowered tumor growth rate and increased the survival time. The data indicate that dietary phytic acid [IP$_6$] has promise as a *pharmacological* [*italics added*] agent in controlling magnesium-ion-mediated tumor promotion. (Jariwalla et al., 1988).

My research on cancer was also published as a chapter entitled "Antineoplastic Action of Inositol Compounds" in the book *Cancer Chemoprevention*, edited by Dr. Lee Wattenberg of the University of Minnesota, and colleagues (Shamsuddin and Sakamoto, 1992), and I refer the reader to that source if he or she is interested.

Boosting Natural Killers

There is yet another important role for IP$_6$ in the regulation of cellular immunity. Natural killer (NK) cells play a central role in various aspects of an organism's defense system. Dr. Abdul Baten, a young man from Bangladesh, who had completed his M.D., and Ph.D. in Moscow, Russia, joined my laboratory with great enthusiasm in 1988. His early work and expertise was on NK cells. Since NK cells are important in getting rid of tumors, he and I investigated whether the anticancer (antineoplastic) action of IP$_6$ was due to the action of NK cells. Using a mouse lymphoma (cancer of the lymph gland) cell line YAC-1 as target cells, the cell-killing ability (cytotoxicity) of mouse spleen NK cells was measured. Mice with carcinogen-induced tumors, treated *in vivo* with IP$_6$, showed greatly enhanced NK activity over the untreated controls. This NK activity correlated with tumor suppression; as the NK activity went up, the incidence of cancer went down (Baten et al., 1989). Similar enhancement of NK activity was also demonstrated when splenocytes from normal mice were treated with IP$_6$ *in vitro* as Dr. Baten and colleagues (including me) showed in 1989.

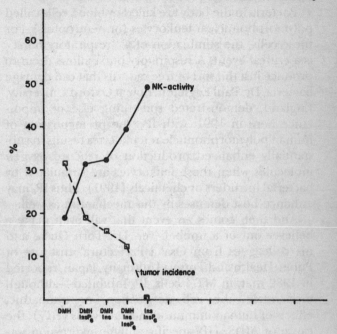

NK-CELL ACTIVITY & TUMOR INCIDENCE (Ins/InsP$_6$)

Figure 4. NK-cell activity and tumor incidence

But what about defenses in the *human* host? Dr. Ivana Vucenik, a researcher from Croatia, became interested in our work. As a hematologist (a scientist who studies the blood), she began investigating human NK activity. In several experiments human NK cells (some of which were from her own blood) were treated with IP$_6$, and as a result, their ability to kill human tumor cells increased. Excited by these results, Ivana decided to continue working on IP$_6$, and as of today she remains as one of my closest collaborators.

Bacteria in the body are killed by blood cells called polymorphonuclear leukocytes (or neutrophils). For these cells, the stimulation of a "respiratory burst" is a critical event. A respiratory burst allows them to produce just the sort of free radicals that can damage bacteria. Dr. Paul Eggleton, now at Oxford University, England, demonstrated something else of importance here in 1991: with IP$_6$, the preincubation of human polymorphonuclear leukocytes results in substantially enhanced production of reactive oxygen molecules when those leukocytes are stimulated by bacterial intruders or chemicals (1991). Thus IP$_6$ may enhance host defenses by this mechanism as well.

And then comes an event that will even make a believer out of a nonbeliever. Dr. Toru Otake and his colleagues from Osaka Prefectural Institute of Public Health and Tottori University, Japan, reported in 1989 that, in MT-4 cells, IP$_6$ inhibited—although moderately—the cell destruction, or cytopathic, effects of human immunodeficiency virus (HIV), the cause of AIDS. HIV-specific antigen expression was also inhibited. Coupled with the facts that IP$_6$ enhances NK-cell activity and the polymorphonuclear cell priming function, it is possible that IP$_6$ may have use in the management of HIV infection and associated immunodeficiency-related problems.

CHAPTER 7

Other Benefits of IP$_6$

Inflammation and Fibrosis

As we now know, asbestos causes fibrosis and cancer in the lungs. Fibrosis is the formation of fibrous tissue as a reparative or reactive process in response to an irritant such as asbestos. It appears that oxidative damage (from superoxide free radicals) plays a crucial role in the early steps in the history of asbestos-induced lung damage. This happens by several mechanisms: by simply causing inflammation, asbestos induces superoxide formation. Also, the iron present in asbestos catalyzes or causes the formation of superoxides through the Fenton reaction, as discussed in Chapter 4.

Because it can remove iron and or inactivate free radicals, IP$_6$ reduces the tissue damage during inflammation. Not only does it reduce the superoxide free radicals, and the resulting DNA damage, IP$_6$ also diminishes the inflammation and resultant fibrosis in the lungs of asbestos-exposed animals. Dr. David W. Kamp and his collaborators (1995a,b) at the Northwestern University Medical School and Veterans Affairs Lakeside Medical Center in Chicago exposed rats to asbestos. Two groups were tested: those with IP$_6$ and a control group without IP$_6$. As expected, asbestos exposure caused a severe inflammatory and fibrotic reaction in the lungs. With IP$_6$ treatment, however, the asbestos-produced inflammation and fibrosis was six- to thirty-fold less. These findings were statistically significant. Based on this information, strategies could be developed to limit asbestos-induced damage in high-risk humans by giving them IP$_6$.

Kidney Stones

Those who have experienced the excruciating pain of kidney stones know what it is like to suffer. Kidney stones, also known as renal calculi or nephrolithiasis, affect approximately 1–5% of the population. These stones are caused by an abnormal accumulation of crystalline substances. Most kidney stones (80–95%) are composed of calcium oxalate and calcium phosphate. Typically, they are located in the calices or pelvis region of the kidneys. They may become lodged in the ureter (which connects the kidney to the bladder), or may be passed to the bladder and voided in the urine. In 50–80% of the individuals who have one episode of kidney stones, there is a recurrence of the painful event.

Patients with kidney stones may experience severe pain or other symptoms that are related to obstruction of the urinary flow or are due to infection. Some more fortunate people may have no symptoms (be asymptomatic), or they may pass the small sand-like stones with relatively little pain. Studies of population groups point to the relationship between diet and kidney stone formation. Since the late nineteenth century, there has been an increased incidence of kidney stones in Europe and North America, with a similar rise in incidence observed in Japan since World War II. Interestingly, such increases in kidney stone incidence coincide with industrial development itself and, along with it, changes in dietary habits.

The population of South Africa presents a good opportunity to examine these issues again. Surveys of South African blacks show a change in their dietary habits when they move from rural to urban areas. For example, the bread eaten by rural South African blacks is either "wholemeal" or brown. With urbanization, however, there is an increasing tendency to eat white bread. Table 2 in Chapter 2 shows that white bread has the least amount of IP$_6$. Table 1 in the same chapter shows that corn has the highest IP$_6$ content of all the cereal grains. It should come as no surprise, then, that the most distinct feature of the diet of rural South African blacks is a high consumption of dried beans and corn. The corn is most commonly eaten in the form of porridge prepared by boiling either home-pounded corn or coarsely ground corn—about 680 grams of corn per person per day! Given the fact that corn may contain up to 6% IP$_6$, that's 40.8 grams of IP$_6$ per day. Dr. Monte Modlin of the Medical School of Cape Town had observed that, in 1970 (and as published in 1980), 5.1 million blacks along with 4.5 million whites, lived in the urban areas. Yet over a 9-year period (1971–

1979), 1 in 510 white patients admitted to the school's main teaching hospital had kidney stones, as opposed to 1 in 44,298 blacks! Even though urban blacks changed their other dietary habits in so far as consuming more meat, they nevertheless continued to eat their traditional corn diet, perhaps accounting for such a low incidence of kidney stones and other diseases.

A high urinary calcium level (hypercalciuria) is common in patients with renal (kidney) calcium stones, and this increases the risk of forming this most common type of stone. It is now known that approximately 1–3% of the total administered IP$_6$ is excreted by human urine. The amount of IP$_6$ in the urine fluctuates between 0.5–5 milligrams per liter of urine with the high level corresponding to increased ingestion of IP$_6$ or diets containing high IP$_6$. Experimentally, IP$_6$ and even IP$_2$ or IP$_3$ are effective in preventing the formation of calcium crystals (Grases et al., 1995, 1996a, 1996b; Modlin, 1980). Thus, logically, a high urinary content of inositol phosphates would effectively inhibit kidney stone formation.

IP$_6$ was used in humans as early as 1958 to prevent and treat kidney stone formation. Dr. Philip H. Henneman and his associates at the Harvard Medical School and Massachusetts General Hospital in Boston successfully used IP$_6$ to treat a condition associated with a high frequency of kidney stones: idiopathic hypercalciuria. In this study, published in the *New England Journal of Medicine*, these investigators selected 24 men, who had normal serum (blood) calcium values, but an increased calcium in the urine (idiopathic hypercalciuria). A total of 8.8 grams of sodium phytate (a salt of IP$_6$) was given daily by mouth in divided doses. IP$_6$ reduced urinary calcium to normal levels. Ten patients received prolonged IP_6 therapy (an average of 24 months). An extended suppression of hypercalciuria was achieved in 9 of those 10 patients, and no further stone growth occurred during therapy in 8 of those patients. IP_6 not only decreased hypercalciuria, but also prevented stone growth and recurrence. Since the alternative treatment—a low-calcium diet (avoidance of milk and cheese) and forcing of fluids (3 to 5 liters a day)—was usually ineffective, IP_6 supplementation was an ideal replacement therapy.

More recently, there seems to be a reemergence of interest in treating and preventing the recurrence of kidney stones by IP_6. Professor F. Grases of the University of the Balearic Islands, off the Spanish coast in the Mediterranean Sea, has recently conducted a study on the treatment of kidney stones by IP_6. He presents his data at *The First International Symposium on Disease Prevention by IP₆ and Other Rice Components* (Kyoto, Japan, June 8–9, 1998) showing a statistically significant decrease in kidney stone formation in 30 patients taking as little as 120 milligrams of IP_6 per day.

A diet containing high amounts of IP_6 (rice bran) has also been used to treat hypercalciuria and kidney stones (Ohkawa et al., 1984). It is definitely easier, to take a small amount of the pure IP_6 in tablets or capsules rather than gorging an enormous quantity of otherwise tasteless rice bran.

Heart Disease

Dietary habits and life-style in Western and more industrialized countries appear to be associated with a high risk for cardiovascular diseases. Population studies have indicated that dietary fiber intake may reduce the risk of coronary heart disease. As blood platelets stick together, they form blood clots, one of the most common causes of subsequent heart attacks. Platelets are irregularly shaped cell fragments made in the bone marrow that travel to the bloodstream. Platelets that group and stick together (or aggregate) form a crucial, early step in the initiation of blood clots (thrombosis) and in complications resulting in cardiovascular diseases such as atherosclerosis, myocardial infarction, and others. Many studies have shown that inhibiting platelet function can prevent blood clots. IP$_6$ is one of the beneficial agents that acts to prevent clots.

My associates, Drs. Ivana Vucenik and John Podczasy, studied the ability of IP$_6$ to inhibit platelet aggregation or clotting. They first used an *in vivo* animal model and then did an experiment with human whole blood *in vitro*. Rats were given 2% IP$_6$ in drinking water for 40 weeks. This would be equal to about 1 to 2 grams (1000 to 2000 milligrams) of IP$_6$ given as an oral dose in a 150-pound human. Platelet aggregation was measured in platelet-rich blood plasma taken from the animals. Rats treated with IP$_6$ showed a 45% inhibition of platelet aggregation.

Measuring platelet aggregation was also performed in human whole blood taken from healthy volunteers. Aggregation of human platelets was initiated by using different substances known to cause "stickiness." This aggregation was significantly reduced by IP$_6$ in a dose-dependent manner. In other words, adding more IP$_6$ produced a larger reduction in clotting. Using IP$_6$ to stop platelet aggregation resulted in 50% lessening to complete elimination of the clotting for all substances tested that produced clots.

This strong antiplatelet activity indicates that IP$_6$ may find its clinical application in reducing the risk of coronary heart diseases, and other diseases that result from blood clots forming and breaking off, such as ischemic stroke.

Heart Attack

The antioxidant function of IP$_6$ makes it ideal for controlling the damage done to the heart muscle (myocardium) during heart attacks. After the onset of a heart attack, there is damage due to *ischemia*, or loss of the blood supply. Blood vessels may be blocked by clots or may temporarily constrict and stop the blood flow. But the heart muscle cells can be saved if the area is successfully filled (reperfused) with oxygenated blood. Obviously, if the lack of blood circulation to the area is cut off for an extended period, an increasing number of heart muscle cells will die. After reperfusion, there will be a mixture of live muscle cells damaged by lack of a blood supply and dead muscle cells. In any event, restoration of arterial blood flow that brings in oxygen is the only way to save the heart muscles from certain death. But it must be done within 6 hours; after that, it is highly unlikely that any muscle cells will be left to salvage.

Paradoxically, reperfusion, and thus the resupply of oxygen, although a well-intentioned effort to save the dying muscle cells, may itself cause more damage. This is called reperfusion injury. Following a brief period of ischemia, reperfusion can completely restore the health of the heart muscles. If the blood supply is not restored within a short period, however, the fresh supply of oxygen causes damage by the free radicals made in the blood. Although oxygen is necessary for life, it can be very toxic when not controlled or kept in check in the body. Recall that oxygen is involved in reactions via oxidation that produce free radicals. An antioxidant is thus a substance that counteracts oxidation and is named for that property. IP$_6$, as we discussed in Chapter 4, has antioxidant properties.

Superoxides, particularly the hydroxyl radical (•OH), have been implicated in the damage done to the myocardium during ischemia and reperfusion. Dr. Parinam S. Rao and colleagues at the Long Island Jewish Medical Center and Albert Einstein College of Medicine in New York, and the University of Connecticut College of Medicine in Farmington, Connecticut, used IP$_6$ to inhibit •OH formation to protect the myocardium from this paradoxical damage (*Annals of Thoracic Surgery*, 1991).

These scientists gave intravenous injections of IP$_6$ in three different dose levels—15 milligrams per kilogram of body weight (mg/kg), 75 mg/kg, and 150 mg/kg to rats 30 minutes before the experiment (equalling 1 gm for a 150-pound human). Ischemia was induced in the rats' hearts after 30 minutes, followed by 30 minutes of reperfusion. A group of rats did not receive IP$_6$; these were the control animals. Rats who received intravenous injections of 75 or 150 mg/kg of IP$_6$ showed protection of the heart muscle from reperfusion injury. This protection could be measured and it was observed that there was improved ventricular function, reduced levels of the key enzyme creatinine kinase (of which an excess indicates heart damage), and decreased lipid peroxidation. Lipid peroxidation is the damage to cellular membranes that is caused by free radicals. "These results suggest the potential use of this antioxidant [IP$_6$] in salvaging the heart from ischemic and reperfusion injury. . . . Phytic acid [IP$_6$], a natural antioxidant, may provide a promising tool for protecting an ischemic heart from reperfusion injury," concluded the authors.

Blood Benefits: More Oxygen and Less Sickle Cell Anemia

The hemoglobin present in our red blood cells binds to oxygen. The oxygen is then delivered to all the cells, or they would die. The ability of the hemoglobin to bind to oxygen, and the ease at which oxygen is released from the hemoglobin, is measured on a graph or chart in the shape of an "S"—the "oxyhemoglobin dissociation curve." A shift of the curve to the right indicates an increase in the ability of oxygen to be released from hemoglobin. When the oxygen is released, there is increased availability of oxygen to the tissues. IP$_6$, when taken in by the red blood cells, results in such a shift (Boucher et al., 1996). So IP$_6$ makes it easier for red blood cells to deliver their oxygen.

Sickle cell disease is a chronic anemia characterized by sickle-shaped red blood cells. Red blood cells are normally slightly oval in shape. The disease results in destruction of red blood cells and is seen almost exclusively in blacks. Variants of the disease are found in people of Mediterranean descent. A very small change in the genetic material (DNA) produces the defect. As a result of this genetic defect, the hemoglobin of sickle cell anemia (called hemoglobin S) has structural abnormalities that cause the red blood cells to sickle or form crescent-like shapes. These inflexible and distorted cells plug small arteries and capillaries, leading to the death of tissues that they service. Furthermore, since the sickled red blood cells are inflexible, they are also fragile and break down easily into small fragments—in a process called hemolysis. Since no effective antisickling agent is currently available, treatment for sickle cell anemia deals only with symptoms such as the pain associated with the disease.

Experimentally, it has been observed that by lowering the concentration of hemoglobin S, sickling can be reduced, allowing the cells to survive for a longer period. By loading IP$_6$ into sickled red blood cells, there is a reduction in hemoglobin S concentration and inhibition of sickling! Therefore, IP$_6$-containing resealed red blood cells have potential in controlling this dreadful disease as well (Boucher et al., 1996). Since dietary IP$_6$ is readily taken up by cells, oral supplementation with IP$_6$ should have a beneficial effect on the sickling of red blood cells.

Cholesterol and Triglycerides

An elevated level of total cholesterol and triglycerides are major risk factors for atherosclerosis and coronary heart disease. In their 1990 work at the Linus Pauling Institute of Science and Medicine, Dr. Raxit Jariwalla and colleagues evaluated the effect of dietary IP$_6$. They found that animals on a cholesterol-enriched diet had their total cholesterol lowered by 19% and triglycerides by 65% when IP$_6$ was added to the diet. The 9% IP$_6$ diet consisted of 8.3% IP$_6$ by weight (calculated), plus an unknown amount of native IP$_6$ present in the rodent chow. A high amount of IP$_6$ was used to more easily demonstrate effects which might also be significant at lower doses. It was not an impractical dose because it is comparable to the therapeutic dose of the prescription drug Questran® (cholestyramine resin), proven effective in lowering death from coronary disease. Effects on levels of zinc and copper were insignificant. Even with a high amount of IP$_6$ as phytate in the diet, these minerals were still available for absorption. In fact, studies have shown that in people with high cholesterol (hypercholesterolemia), levels of zinc are too high compared with copper. IP$_6$ actually normalizes the zinc to copper ratio. This lowering of zinc occurred only in animals fed a high-cholesterol diet, not those on a normal diet. So IP$_6$ merely restored serum mineral balance in animals with high cholesterol. In addition, the breakdown products of IP$_6$ (the lower IPs) have been shown in animal studies to remove calcification of arteries. Such effects as we have shown may find use in the clinical management of high blood cholesterol (hyperlipidemia) and diabetes.

CHAPTER 8

And That's Not All

Defusing Liver Cancer Cells

Liver cancer, also called hepatocellular carcinoma, is common in China, and other areas of the world where hepatitis B virus is prevalent. In North America, the incidence is 3 to 7 cases per 100,000 people. Rather than hepatitis, however, this cancer is associated with cirrhosis of the liver caused by alcohol, excess iron, and other toxins. Liver cancer is a deadly, malignant disease with an extremely poor prognosis. Death usually occurs within six months of diagnosis. Many therapies have been proposed, but there is still uncertainty about their effectiveness.

Dr. Zhenshu Zhang from Nanfang Hospital of the First PLA Medical College in Guangzhou, China, came to my laboratory in the summer of 1997. He did not have any specific project in mind. After a brief discussion, I came to learn that in China, and specifically in his hospital, they attempt to treat liver cancer in humans by injecting alcohol directly within the tumors. I thought that we could try something similar. I wanted to study whether IP_6 had potential in the treatment of liver cancer. In preparation for such a mode of treatment, we performed a pilot study to test whether IP_6 would suppress the formation and growth of human cancer cells. But before we embarked on the study—which not only would be costly in terms of money but could also entail unnecessary use of research animals—we decided to test whether or not the human cancer cells would be responsive to IP_6. For if they were unresponsive *in vitro* (in the laboratory), then we would not go ahead with an animal experiment. We thus took human liver cancer cells (hepatocellular carcinoma HepG2) and grew this cell line in the laboratory with or without IP_6.

When we treated the human cancer cells with IP_6, we found that the growth of these cells was inhibited. The growth inhibition was dose-dependent, meaning that as more IP_6 was added, the cells were inhibited more and more. These cancer cells were highly sensitive to the cancer-fighting ability of IP_6, and so much so that the growth of the cancerous cells became completely inhibited.

We then did an experiment where we took human liver cancer cells and injected them into mice. In 71% of the mice that did not first receive IP_6 before being exposed to the cancer, a solid tumor growth was observed. In those mice receiving the same number of HepG2 liver cancer cells that had been pretreated *in vitro* with IP_6 for 48 hours before being injected, no tumor was found. So exposing the cancerous tumor cells to IP_6 had somehow stopped them from out-of-control growth and from forming a tumor. For mice with established tumors, IP$_6$ also had beneficial results. When the tumors reached 8–10 millimeters in diameter (about a basketball-sized tumor for us), injection of IP$_6$ was made into the tumor for 12 consecutive days. The tumor weight in the IP$_6$-treated mice was 3.4-fold less than that in control mice who didn't receive any IP$_6$.

The most intriguing finding in this experiment lay here: a single treatment of cancer cells with IP$_6$ resulted in complete loss of the ability of these cells to form tumors. On the other hand, the untreated cells formed tumors in the mice. Even more exciting was the effect on preexisting liver cancers themselves. When they were treated directly with IP$_6$, they regressed. This experiment showed that IP$_6$ can be used to treat highly malignant hepatocellular carcinoma as well.

Rhabdomyosarcoma: A Malignant Childhood Cancer

Rhabdomyosarcomas are tumors made up of cells that resemble primitive skeletal muscle-forming cells, and they exert a very aggressive behavior. These types of tumors are the most common soft tissue sarcomas in children and young adults, usually appearing within the first two decades of life. As aggressive cancers, they are usually treated with a combination of surgery, radiation, and chemotherapy. However, they do not respond to any conventional therapy in patients with cancers that have spread (metastases). There is thus an urgent need for new therapies for these cancers.

In Chapter 5 we discussed how IP$_6$ induces maturation (differentiation) of human colon, prostate, and breast cancer cells. Since rhabdomyosarcoma cells are primitive or immature, my colleague Dr. Vucenik, in collaboration with Dr. Thea Kalebic and coworkers (1997), wanted to test whether IP_6 would cause this human cancer cell line (RD cells) to mature as well. The RD cells originally came from a human rhabdomyosarcoma tumor.

We first looked at the effects of IP_6 on human rhabdomyosarcoma in cell culture (in a laboratory dish). We took some RD cancer cells and exposed them to different concentrations of IP_6 continuously for 5 days. We also exposed some RD cells to different concentrations of IP_6 for 6, 12, 24, or 72 hours. Then we removed IP_6 and allowed the cells to continue to grow. This treatment was given every other day. We also took some RD cancer cells and treated them with IP_6 for 3 days, stopped and let them grow (for about 3 days) without IP_6, and then gave them another 3 days of IP_6 treatment. Our results for the RD cells treated continuously for 7 days showed that IP_6 suppresses the growth of the human rhabdomyosarcoma cell line (RD) *in vitro* in a dose-dependent fashion (higher doses result in more suppression). The RD cells that were treated with IP_6 every other day for 6, 12, or 24 hours yielded a similar response as continuous treatment of RD cells for 5 days.

Results with the RD cells treated for 3 days with IP_6, then 3 days off IP_6, followed by another 3 days on IP_6 were as follows: When IP_6 was removed after 3 days, the RD cells began to grow again, but not as fast as those that had never been exposed to IP_6. When IP_6 was added back (a second exposure), the RD cells again decreased in growth rate. What is important about this experiment is that the RD cells did not develop resistance to IP$_6$. They were still responsive to the growth-diminishing effects of IP$_6$ when exposed the second time. For many conventional treatments of cancer cells, such as chemotherapy, the cells can become resistant to the effects of the drug. This did not happen with IP$_6$. Also important was the fact that the RD cells did not grow well in the culture dish after IP$_6$ treatment. Cancer cells that are healthy and aggressive form colonies of cells in culture dishes. The colonies grow and run into each other, filling up the whole dish with wall-to-wall cancer cells. They may even pile up on top of one another and usually don't stop growing until all the nutrients in the culture medium are exhausted. The ability of RD cells to form colonies decreased with increasing concentrations of IP$_6$ added to the culture medium.

Shape (or morphological) changes were particularly obvious after exposure of cancerous RD cells to IP$_6$. Untreated cancerous RD cells are typically small, spindle-shaped cells attached to the bottom of the culture dish in an irregular arrangement, and with no evidence of skeletal muscle maturation (differentiation). In contrast, the appearance of the cells changed following a second or third 3-day treatment with IP$_6$. Exposure of RD cells to IP$_6$ led to differentiation, which is a normal step for noncancerous cells. The cells became larger and made higher levels of muscle-specific actin, a protein that is specifically present in normally differentiated skeletal muscle cells. Cancerous RD cells would not make this protein. This changed appearance of RD cells toward normal shape and function remained stable for at least 3–4 passages of cells into a new culture medium (material on which cells grow). So even in this short-term experiment, there was a favorable outcome with IP_6

We also wanted to see the effects of IP_6 on the human cancer cells if they were in a live organism. Putting human cancer cells into an animal and treating the animal with the agent that is designed to kill or stop the cancer cells is an accepted method of testing. It is done before the anticancer substance is given to humans with cancer. In this experiment, we used mice with no thymus gland (athymic mice) to determine the effect of IP_6 on the tumor-forming capacity of RD cells. The thymus is an important part of the immune system. Having animals without a thymus would allow us to transplant human tumor cells in them, so that we could test the effectiveness of anticancer agents against *human* cancer in an animal. Each mouse thus received viable (live) human RD cells, injected under the skin into the lower back region. Then IP_6 was injected around the tumor. The amount of IP_6 given to the mice was 40 milligrams per kilogram of weight. This would be equal to about 2,800 mg (about 2.8 grams) of IP_6 for a 150-pound human. The treatment was started 2 days after injection of tumor cells, and was continued every other day, 3 times weekly, either for 2 weeks (Experiment 1) or for 5 weeks (Experiment 2). The control animals received only the tumor cells. All animals received proper care and maintenance in accordance with institutional guidelines for humane treatment. Tumor growth was monitored twice weekly and mice were checked for any other abnormalities.

A significant decrease of tumor growth was observed in animals treated with IP_6. The treatment with IP_6 caused a decrease in tumor incidence and suppressed growth of tumors. While all the animals that did not receive IP$_6$ developed tumors, only 40% of the IP$_6$-treated animals from Experiment 1 and 20% of IP$_6$-treated animals from Experiment 2 produced tumors. Tumors, if any, were 25 to 49 times smaller in IP$_6$-treated animals, when compared to untreated controls. Also the tumors that did appear in IP$_6$-treated animals were at 25 days after tumor injection as opposed to 10 days in untreated animals. These results, showing a significant decrease of tumor growth, were consistent in two independent experiments. The tumors found in IP$_6$-treated animals and control animals looked the same. The tumors in the IP$_6$-treated group, however, were found to have a lower mitotic rate. This means that the tumor cells were dividing and multiplying at a slower rate. The results of these experiments show that IP$_6$ is an effective inhibitor of tumor growth and an inducer of maturation in human RD cells.

Consistent with the *in vitro* (cell culture) observations, IP$_6$ suppressed RD cell growth *in vivo* in the athymic mice. As mentioned above, when compared to controls, IP$_6$-treated mice produced 25-fold smaller tumors, as observed after 2 weeks of treatment. In a second experiment, of 4 weeks of IP$_6$ treatment, a 49-fold reduction in tumor size was observed. Under the microscope, no evidence of tumor cell breakdown (necrosis) was observed, confirming all the previous studies that IP$_6$ does not kill tumor cells. This may be a good way to stop cancer cells. In some cases, chemotherapeutic drugs or radiation treatments cause tumors to undergo necrosis too quickly and the patient's body has to get rid of a large amount of toxic tumor debris and dead cancer cells. IP$_6$, on the other hand, only stops cell growth, and is noncytotoxic, yet it suppresses the tumors by 25- to 49-fold!

This dramatic effect in live animals suggests that IP_6 may affect the growth of human rhabdomyosarcomas in the same manner.

These experiments also indicate that amounts of IP_6 higher than in the normal body are needed to combat cancer cells—meaning that supplementation is necessary. Together with the finding that the cancer cells do not become resistant to IP_6, these studies suggest a great potential of IP_6 as a new approach to conventional therapy of rhabdomyosarcoma and other related tumors.

Colon Cancer: IP_6 vs. Green Tea

For those who are tea drinkers and are rushing to gulp down that extra cup because you have heard that drinking green tea may prevent cancer, here is some news. As you may already have heard, it has recently been suggested that green tea may be beneficial in reducing the risk of stomach and skin cancer. To test whether it may be beneficial in colon cancer as well, in 1997 Drs. Anjana Challa and D. Ramkishan Rao at the Alabama A & M University and Dr. Bandaru S. Reddy at the American Health Foundation, New York, investigated its efficacy in reducing the risk of colon cancer in an experimental rat model.

Since an investigation of the final tumor incidence takes a long time and, consequently, is more expensive, it has become a routine to check for cancer markers to measure the benefit (or lack thereof) of a test agent. These markers appear before the cancer becomes detectable; thus they are also called "intermediate biomarkers." In the colon, the glands or crypts in the wall of the colon are normally test-tube shaped. Early during cancer formation, these crypts lose their regular test-tube shape, become distended, have more cells, and are therefore abnormal. Conglomerations of several such crypts are called "Aberrant Crypt Foci" or ACF for short. These aberrant crypts are precancerous and therefore have a high risk of becoming cancer.

Using ACF as the intermediate biomarker, Drs. Challa, Rao, and Reddy tested whether green tea has any preventative effect on colon cancer. They compared the efficacy effectiveness of IP$_6$ with that of green tea. Green tea was given in drinking water (0, 1, 2%) to one group of rats, and the same level of IP$_6$ (0, 1, 2%) was given to a second group of rats but in the feed. Another group of rats received both green tea in the water and IP$_6$ in the feed.

The authors concluded that green tea had a marginal effect that was not statistically significant. On the other hand, the reduction in the number of ACF by IP$_6$ was marked and statistically significant. When IP$_6$ was given along with green tea, the results, as you can predict, were better. Thus not only was IP$_6$ by itself beneficial, but it worked synergistically with green tea.

How did the IP$_6$ work to reduce the risk of cancer? Glutathione S-transferase (GST) is a key enzyme responsible for detoxifying various chemicals that enter the body, including cancer-causing agents. It is desirable that these toxic chemicals be destroyed so as to protect ourselves, and that is what GST does. Therefore, substances that increase the activity of GST would likely protect us better. These researchers thus tested the effects of IP$_6$ and green tea on the enzyme GST. While green tea had no effect on the level of GST, feeding 2% IP$_6$ (equivalent to 1–2 grams of IP_6 in an oral dose for humans) resulted in a statistically significant increase in GST activity in the liver of those rats. Thus, IP_6 not only reduced the number of the precancerous ACFs, but enhanced the body's ability to destroy cancer-causing chemicals by increasing GST activity.

Safety of IP_6

IP_6 is a very safe nutrient and its use is not associated with any significant adverse effects. In experiments conducted by my group, there was no significant toxic effect on body weight, serum mineral content, or any pathological changes of consequence in rats given IP_6. Two strains of rats from both genders—either male F344 rats or female Sprague-Dawley rats—were observed by us for 40 weeks (Shamsuddin and Sakamoto, 1992; Vucenik et al., 1993). Although short-term studies have shown that high levels of IP_6 reduce absorption of calcium, with continued intake of diets rich in IP_6, calcium absorption increases to normal levels (Bhaskaram and Reddy, 1979). In fact, these researchers had shown that following long-term intake of a diet rich in IP_6 (45.4 milligrams per kilogram or over 3 grams), there was no significant toxicity; indeed, calcium absorption had improved. Some studies have shown that IP_6 binding to minerals can prevent absorption of these minerals from the diet. Graf and Eaton (1990), however, have shown that IP_6 binding to minerals is easily disrupted, leaving the mineral free to be absorbed. These researchers also have shown that minerals can be even more available to the body in the presence of IP_6 (1984). Jariwalla and colleagues (1988) also reported that rats with tumors fed up to 12% IP$_6$ as phytate (equivalent to a dose of 6 to 12 grams in a 150-pound human) caused no discomfort or toxicity. These researchers also pointed out that none of the other forms of inositol phosphates resulting from metabolism of IP$_6$ were toxic or strongly reactive as well.

Of particular note in the evaluation of IP$_6$ safety is the work of Henneman and colleagues from Massachusetts General Hospital and Harvard Medical School, who described their studies with humans in the *New England Journal of Medicine* in 1958. They administered pure IP$_6$ orally to 35 patients at a dose of 8.8 g/day (in divided doses) for an average of 24 months. These patients had high calcium content in the urine (hypercalciuria), a condition frequently found in patients with kidney stones. Not only did IP$_6$ reduce the episodes of urinary stones in these patients, a long-term follow-up study of 10 patients showed no untoward side effects; the reduction in hypercalciuria and prevention of stone recurrence were rather the benefits. In follow-up studies of patients with hypercalciuria, T. Ohkawa and colleagues (1984), treated patients with 10 grams of rice bran (high in IP$_6$) for up to 2 years. There was no decrease, significant or otherwise, in blood serum calcium, phosphate, or magnesium, again dispelling concern about the mineral-chelating effect of IP$_6$. There is other verification of the lack of effect on mineral metabolism as given below.

". . . concern has been expressed that phytic acid [IP$_6$] intake, and insoluble fiber intake in general, might have adverse effects owing to the *alleged* [italics mine] lower availability of essential micronutrients and, in particular, minerals like magnesium, zinc, and calcium. This fear is based on historic observations in areas like Iran, where the traditional daily nutritional regime involved chiefly the consumption of high phytate fiber pita bread without many other foods serving as sources of minerals, vitamins, and like essential micronutrients. This kind of unbalanced nutrition has led to poor development and growth in children and resulted in dwarfism. However, in other parts of the world, particularly in the Western world, with the general availability of a great variety of many foods, including fruits and vegetables as well as meats and fish, as sources of essential minerals and vitamins, *there is no fear of mineral and vitamin deficiencies, even in the presence of an adequate intake of cereal fiber and even phytate IP_6,* [italics added]. The Finnish people have a low colon cancer rate and a lower breast cancer rate than Europeans and Americans, generally because of a high cereal insoluble fiber intake, and these populations do not display any signs of mineral and vitamin deficiencies leading to abnormal growth and development (Weisburger et al., 1993)."

And:

"In view of the recent evidence that . . . phytic acid (IP_6) is anti-neoplastic it may be that consumption of undegraded phytates should be encouraged notwithstanding the nutritional implications (Iqbal et al., 1994).

If safety had ever been an issue, the following information about the use of IP$_6$ as a diagnostic and research tool should eliminate any doubts completely and irrevocably. In imaging of the liver and spleen for diagnostic radiology, the patient is given a radioactive "cocktail" so that the organ of interest will "light up" on the x-ray or other detection device. Many substances have been tested to carry radioactive compounds into the body, such as ^{99m}-technetium (Tc). Most of these carrier substances take only 10-13% of the radioactive particles to the target tissue, resulting in poor images. To alleviate this problem, Dr. G. Subramanian and coworkers at the Upstate Medical Center, Syracuse, NY, developed the protocol for using IP$_6$ as a carrier for ^{99m}Tc. "The acute intravenous toxicity of this compound is very low. . . . Thus, ^{99m}Tc-Sn-phytate appears promising as a nontoxic agent . . . [Subramanian et al., 1973]."

Since then, the use of IP$_6$ in diagnostic radiology has been extensive throughout the world (Chang et al., 1996; Efrati et al., 1996). "We use the radiocolloid ^{99m}Tc phytate [IP$_6$] routinely during liver scanning of almost all inpatients with liver disease," states Dr. S. Shiomi and colleagues of Osaka City Medical University, Japan (Shiomi et al., 1996). Not only is it easy to prepare the solution for application, but the imaging is also reported to be superior, and it offers additional advantage in prognosis (forecast of the probable course and/or outcome of a disease) of patients: ". . . hepatic imaging with ^{99m}Tc-phytate, in addition to its diagnostic value, also contains valuable prognostic information in patients with cirrhosis" (Picard et al., 1990).

* * *

In the search for a "simple, effective, *safe, and well-tolerated* [italics mine] contrast agent . . . as a bowel marker in magnetic resonance (MR) imaging," Dr. E. C. Unger and collaborators at the University of Arizona Health Sciences Center in Tucson (1993) investigated the use of iron-IP_6 in human volunteers. They demonstrated that iron and IP_6 mixed well with food stuff, functioned as an effective gastrointestinal MR contrast agent, and significantly improved the bowel contrast.

Drs. S. K. Chung, H. H. Kim, and Y. W. Bahk of Catholic University Medical College of Seoul, Korea (1997) have extended the diagnostic use of ^{99m}Tc-IP_6 to aerosol ventilation scanning of the lung. Seven patients with bronchial obstruction and one with stenosis (narrowing) were given the ^{99m}Tc-IP_6 aerosol generated by a nebulizer (the mixture was sprayed into the lung). The ventilation scan showed characteristic intense aerosol deposition in the bronchial segments immediately proximal to (next to) the obstruction or constriction, once again demonstrating not only the utility, but also the safety of IP_6.

CHAPTER 9

Inositol: Mother of IP$_6$

A Unique B Vitamin

Inositol, although not officially a B vitamin, is recognized as part of the B complex group. There is no RDA for inositol, but most people get about 1000 milligrams a day from their food. Inositol is found in food in two forms. IP$_6$ in the fiber of plant foods is turned into inositol when good bacteria in your intestines digest it. You also get inositol in the form of myo-inositol. While *myo-* means "muscle," this form is found both in plant and in animal foods. Good sources include organ meats, citrus fruits, nuts, beans, and whole grains.

The word *complex* indicates that all eleven of the B vitamins are commonly found together in foods. Inositol is water soluble, and is not stored very well in the body. (Fat-soluble vitamins tend to be stored in fatty tissue in the body.) Thus, an intake of inositol is needed daily to support its many functions. Deficiencies of inositol or other B vitamins may occur fairly easily, especially during times of fasting or weight-loss diets or with diets that include substantial amounts of refined and processed food, sugar, or alcohol. Caffeine in large quantities may create an inositol shortage. Heavy drinkers of coffee, tea, cocoa, and other caffeine-containing substances may therefore need additional amounts.

Inositol is an important component of biological membranes, such as those that surround cells. Inositol is part of phosphatidylinositol, a phospholipid. Phospholipids are important in keeping cell membranes fluid or soft, which is essential for allowing nutrients into cells and waste products out. The neurotransmitters serotonin (elevated by the drug Prozac™ and the herb St. John's wort) and acetylcholine both require phosphatidylinositol for proper functioning.

The *Physicians' Desk Reference Family Guide to Nutrition and Health* (1995) says that inositol has not been found to be toxic at any dosage level. In fact, according to Michael Lesser, M.D., "as much as 50 grams (50,000 milligrams) has been taken by mouth with no ill effect." Dr. Lesser indicates that inositol has a mild antianxiety effect, similar to that of mild tranquilizers, but without the side effects. This may be related to its interaction with serotonin or other neurotransmitters. Inositol can also lower blood pressure, help remove fatty deposits from the liver, and can naturally induce sleep. By assisting in the proper utilization of fat and cholesterol, inositol lowers blood cholesterol levels, thus protecting the arteries and heart. Inositol is also found in high quantities in the brain.

Table 6.
Natural Sources of Inositol

Beans, dried
Calves' liver
Cantaloupe
Citrus fruit, except lemons
Garbanzo beans (chickpeas)
Lecithin granules
Lentils
Nuts
Oats
Pork
Rice
Veal
Wheat germ
Whole-grain products

Inositol has a carbohydrate structure identical to IP$_6$, minus the phosphates and, as noted in Table 6, can be found in animal and plant tissue. It is estimated, as mentioned above, that adults consume approximately 1 gram of inositol per day. Human diets of animal and plant sources contain inositol in its free form; cow's milk contains approximately 30–80 milligrams of inositol per liter. Not only has inositol been determined to pose no dietary health hazard, it is normally added to infant formulas at a concentration of 0.01%. Animal products such as fish, poultry, and beef have inositol as inositol-containing phospholipids, or as inositol hexaphosphate (IP$_6$); the latter is the most important source of inositol in food from plant sources. The enzyme phytase is found in plants, animals, and fungi. Present in the intestinal mucosa (lining) of many animals including rats, calves, chickens, and pigs, it removes the phosphates from IP$_6$ in a time-dependent manner. This results in the formation of free inositol, and the lower phosphorylated forms of inositol: IP$_{1-5}$. Although this happens in experimental animals, such may not be the case in humans, for the phytase activity in our gut is thirty-fold less than that in rats.

Inositol is also made in the body from glucose (in normal human kidneys) at the rate of about 4 grams per day. Glucose with 6 phosphate groups attached (glucose-6-phosphate) is converted to inositol-1-phosphate and finally to inositol. Experimental studies have demonstrated that approximately 50% of the free inositol in the rabbit's brain is made from glucose right in the brain; the other 50% coming from the blood. Inositol is broken down (degraded) to carbon dioxide (CO_2) by the kidneys.

Dietary inositol deficiency is reported to cause decreased growth rate and loss of hair (alopecia) in mice. In culturing human and animal cells in the laboratory, it is essential that inositol be added to the growth media, for without it the cells do not grow. Thus it is an essential growth factor. In normal humans, free inositol is found in the blood plasma. Mammalian (including human) semen is rich in free inositol, containing several fold higher levels than in blood plasma. High concentrations of inositol are found in the testes and epididymis (which transports and stores sperm). The epididymis also contains a higher level of inositol than in the testes. The levels of free inositol in brain and cerebrospinal spinal fluid (the bath water of the brain and spinal cord) are also higher than that in the blood plasma.

Health Benefits of Inositol

Fat metabolism. Dietary inositol, like choline, is a lipotropic agent, meaning that it reduces the amount of fat in the liver. Animals fed diets lacking inositol develop low levels of cholesterol (hypocholesterolemia), and excessive amounts of fat in the liver and in the inner layer of bowel wall (intestinal lipodystrophy). Levels of cholesterol that are too low (in some studies with values of less than 150 milligrams/deciliter) result in the weakening of blood vessel walls, thus increasing the risk of stroke. Cholesterol, we must remember, is also needed in the cell membrane of all cells. With their resulting weight loss, these deficient animals eventually die prematurely. Treatment with inositol, however, can reverse the intestinal lipodystrophy as well as excessive fat in the liver. Excessive liver fat can also be reduced by IP$_6$ treatment, as T. Katayama found in 1995. In this case, rats were fed a high-sugar diet which resulted in increases in liver weight (due to fat accumulation), triglyceride, and cholesterol levels. Addition of inositol (as phytate) to the diet, lowered all these values.

Diabetes. The metabolism of inositol is altered in diabetes mellitus, kidney diseases, and several other diseases. Inositol deficiency within the cells in patients with diabetes is implicated in the development of various complications of diabetes, such as altered sensations in the nerves of the feet and hands (peripheral neuropathy), cataract and retinal damage, and early derangements of kidney functions (diabetic nephropathy).

In experimentally induced diabetes mellitus in animals, the free inositol level in the peripheral nerves is reduced. This is correlated with problems in muscle movement and sensation via nerve impulses traveling more slowly, and known as decreased motor nerve conduction velocity. Insulin treatment prevents this decrease in inositol level in the cells and reverses the impaired nerve conduction velocity. Taking dietary supplementation of inositol, which elevates plasma inositol levels, has also been proven beneficial in alleviating the depressed motor nerve conduction. Also, there are certain conditions such as chronic renal failure where the level of blood plasma inositol may be as high as seven-fold more than normal. These high levels in the blood are an indication that the kidneys are not working properly and that inositol is not getting to the cells that use it. Such a rise in plasma inositol level may be related to a depression in nerve conduction velocity as well (Holub, 1986).

In any event, dosages of inositol, ranging from 0.5 gram twice a day to 3 grams a day have been given to patients with diabetic neuropathy, and results to date support that oral supplementation of inositol may be of benefit in the prevention and treatment of neural complications of diabetes mellitus.

Birth defects. Diabetes mellitus is one of the most common diseases affecting the mother that results in congenital malformations of the baby that are incompatible with life. Such birth defects account for approximately 40% of perinatal deaths among children of diabetic mothers. The incidence of this abnormality in the embryo (embryopathy) in diabetic mothers is four to five times higher than that in the general population. Congenital malformations occur during early pregnancy when the organs are being formed and when the pregnancy is hardly recognizable. The mechanism for causing malformations in experimental diabetic pregnancy (in animals) was found by several researchers to include generation of free oxygen radicals and alterations in the levels of inositol in the embryo. As for free radicals, antioxidants are the logical antidote. In experimental systems, it has been demonstrated that by increasing the glucose concentration in the embryo, the inositol level is lowered. On the other hand, inositol supplementation restores the concentrations to normal levels with a significant decrease in the rate of malformation. This restoration in inositol levels is believed to reflect the restored membrane integrity. Although IP$_6$, which has antioxidant function, has not been tested, other antioxidants and inositol "offer significant promise for the future in possibly serving as a pharmacological prophylaxis against diabetic embryopathy" (Reece, and Eriksson, 1996).

Dr. Reece and his colleagues further demonstrated that with dietary inositol supplementation, the incidence of neural tube defect, a malformation in the early embryo that results in birth defects primarily involving the brain and other parts of the nervous system, can be reduced from 20.4% to 9.5%; this decrease being statistically significant. ". . . data demonstrate that *myo*-inositol [inositol] supplementation reduces the incidence of diabetic embryopathy and may serve as a pharmacologic prophylaxis against diabetes-induced congenital malformations" (Reece, et al., 1997).

Psychiatric diseases. Several psychiatric diseases have been treated with inositol. These include clinical depression, panic disorder, and obsessive-compulsive disorder. The inositol level in brain cells is reduced in a variety of neuropsychiatric disorders. It has been found that the inositol level in the cerebrospinal fluid is decreased in patients with depression. Dr. G. Agam and his coworkers at Soroka Medical Center, Beer-Sheva, Israel, demonstrated that administration of inositol into the ventricles of the brain reverses seizures in experimental animals. Large doses of inositol given via injection into the body cavity raises the low level of inositol in the cerebrospinal fluid and can also reverse experimental seizures. "Demonstration that inositol enters the brain after peripheral administration provides a basis for possible pharmacological intervention in psychiatric disorders," the authors conclude (Agam et al., 1994).

Two clinical trials have shown that large amounts of inositol can improve certain psychiatric disorders such as mental depression. A double-blind controlled clinical trial (the type of study accepted by conventional scientists and physicians worldwide) was performed at the Ben Gurion University of the Negev, by the Israeli Ministry of Health, Mental Health Center, on clinically depressed patients. When 28 depressed patients were given 12 grams of inositol a day, a statistically significant overall benefit was found for inositol treatment as compared to the placebo control (the group that did not receive the inositol). This improvement occurred as early as week 4 on the Hamilton Depression Scale, the standard measure to assess the effectiveness of an antidepressant substance (Levine, 1997).

Since many antidepressants are also effective in panic disorder, Dr. J. Levine studied the effect of inositol treatment on 21 patients with this disorder in a double-blind, placebo-controlled, random-assignment crossover treatment trial (another acceptable study design) using 12 grams of inositol per day. Some of these patients had agoraphobia, an extreme fear of open spaces. After 4 weeks of treatment with inositol, the frequency and severity of panic attacks and the severity of agoraphobia was reduced with inositol treatment as opposed to the placebo control; the reduction was statistically significant.

In another study, thirteen patients with obsessive-compulsive disorder were treated with 18 grams of inositol or placebo per day for 6 weeks in a double-blind controlled crossover trial. Here, too, inositol reduced the symptoms of obsessive-compulsive disorder, as scored on the Yale-Brown Obsessive-Compulsive Scale with good statistical significance when compared to the placebo control.

No significant change in the blood tests for blood (hematologic) disorders, and kidney or liver function tests were noted with these treatments, much less any toxicity. "The authors conclude that inositol is effective in depression, panic, and obsessive-compulsive disorder, a spectrum of disorders responsive to serotonin reuptake inhibitors" (Fux et al., 1996). Prozac is an example of a serotonin reuptake inhibitor.

Liver diseases. Dr. Tetsuyuki Katayama of Hiroshima University, Japan, has shown that dietary supplementation with inositol or IP$_6$ decreases the amount of fat in the liver and the blood (Katayama, 1995). Similar conclusions were derived by other investigators. Dr. Raxit Jariwalla, then at the Linus Pauling Institute of Science and Medicine in Palo Alto, California, also reported that addition of IP$_6$ reduced serum cholesterol and triglyceride levels in rats, and these were statistically significant results (Jariwalla et al., 1990). What Dr. Katayama also found is that these levels are not lowered in normal otherwise healthy animals, but only in animals in whom the levels are induced to be high.

As you know, high levels of serum lipids increase the risk for atherosclerosis. By the same token, increased fat in the liver is an early stage of more serious problems such as cirrhosis. Thus the relevance of this is quite substantial insofar as prevention and perhaps treatment of cardiovascular diseases and fatty liver are concerned.

Patients with severe liver disease resulting in failure of liver functions undergo a condition called *hepatic encephalopathy,* or hepatic coma. This is characterized by personality changes; impaired consciousness, ranging from drowsiness to coma; and other symptoms. Inositol is found to be depleted in the brain of these patients (Lien et al., 1994).

Cancer prevention. I first demonstrated that inositol alone or in combination with IP$_6$ could prevent the formation and incidence of several cancers in experimental animals. Those in prevention of soft tissue, colon, and mammary cancers will be described elsewhere. Herein I will describe its usefulness against lung cancer.

Dr. Lee W. Wattenberg of the University of Minnesota, Minneapolis, has been studying the preventive action of lung cancer in various experimental models. Benzo[a]pyrene and 4-(methylnitrosamino)-1-(3-pyridyl)-1-butanone are two of the major chemicals thought to cause lung cancer. Dr. Wattenberg and his colleague have shown that inositol prevents the benzo[a]pyrene-induced lung tumor formation in female A/J mice (Estensen and Wattenberg, 1993). This treatment was effective even when it was started

1 week after the carcinogen was given (i.e., during the postinitiation phase). Suffice it to mention here that if inositol treatment was started 2 weeks prior to carcinogen treatment and continued through the duration of the experiment, it reduced lung tumor formation by 64%. Dr. Wattenberg further extended his studies to test the efficacy of inositol inhibition of lung tumor induced by yet another carcinogen, 4-(methylnitrosamino)-1-(3-pyridyl)-1-butanone.

They also tested the ability of a synthetic steroid (dexamethasone) to inhibit tumor formation with a combination of inositol + dexamethasone. Inositol reduced the tumor formation by 46%, whereas dexamethasone reduced it by 41% and the combination by 71%. Dexamethasone, however, produces adverse effects associated with steroids such as cataract, glaucoma, and the promotion of infection. Drs. Wattenberg and Estensen conclude, " . . . *myo*-inositol and dexamethasone inhibit pulmonary adenoma formation resulting from exposures to two major pulmonary carcinogens, B(*a*)P and 4-(methyl-nitrosamino)-1-(3-pyridyl)-1-butanone" (Wattenberg and Estensen, 1996).

CHAPTER 10

An Anticancer Cocktail: IP_6 + Inositol

Making a Good Thing Better

As I stated earlier, my hypothesis about IP_6 concerns the following. IP_6 undergoes dephosphorylation. This means that an enzyme (a phosphatase) removes phosphate (P) molecules, resulting in a pool of inositol phosphates: IP_{1-5}. The IP_3 that is produced is central in sending chemical messages (signal transduction) and in other cell functions such as division. So IP_6 could enter into the intracellular inositol phosphate pool and cause tumor suppression through its conversion to lower inositol phosphates such as IP_3.

I had also hypothesized that inositol could also become phosphorylated by enzymes called kinases. In this case, phosphate groups are added resulting in the higher inositol phosphates such as IP_{1-6}, but most importantly IP_3.

If inositol is then added to IP_6 and given as a nutritional cocktail, it would allow the newly released phosphates from IP_6 to be captured by the inositol that's nearby. Therefore, delivering IP_6 + inositol seems to increase availability of lower inositol phosphates, most importantly IP_3, as shown in the following reaction:

$$IP_6 + inositol \rightarrow 2\ IP_3$$

If, indeed, IP_3 is involved in the transmission of signals from the growth factors on the cell's exterior to the nucleus inside the cell, and if IP_3 acts in cell division, too much of this signal may cause an overload. The excess may shut down cell proliferation and cell growth. Furthermore, because inositol phosphates are found everywhere and are common molecules involved in signal transduction in most mammalian cell systems, I also hypothesized that the anticancer action of inositol phosphates would be observed in different cells and tissue systems. You have already read about the anticancer function of IP_6 against various tumors and they are summarized in Table 5 in Chapter 6. What follows are examples of how the combination treatment is also better than just inositol or IP_6 alone in several different cancers.

It was once said that "research is 99% drudgery and misery and 1% eureka!" Getting that 1% reward can take a long time. When I had proposed these hypotheses back in the mid-1980s, inositol had not as yet been shown to be converted to IP_6. It was not until 1990 that L. R. Stephens and R. F. Irvine of Cambridge, U.K. showed that the conversion does take place, for their purposes, in the slime mold, *Dictyostelium* (remember we said inositol and IP_6 are everywhere). Other researchers commented that such a conversion had not been shown in mammalian cells. But that is how research evolves from a hypothesis. *Merriam-Webster's Collegiate Dictionary* defines hypothesis as "a *tentative assumption* [italics mine] made in order to draw out and test its logical or empirical [experimental] consequences. . . . [The word] HYPOTHESIS implies insufficient evidence to provide more than a tentative explanation." So a hypothesis is a door we open to advance to further knowledge. It often takes longer for minds to be opened. With perseverance and good research, however, hypotheses become known as facts.

Cancer-Fighting Combination

Mammary tumors. In Table 7, the results of experiments in my laboratory with a rat mammary tumor model are shown. The rats were induced to have mammary tumors by exposing them to the cancer-causing agent, DMBA (7,12-dimethylbenz[a]-anthracene). Starting at 2 weeks prior to tumor induction with DMBA, the drinking water of the rats was supplemented with either IP$_6$, inositol, or IP$_6$ + inositol. The DMBA-only group did not have any inositol or IP$_6$ in the drinking water and therefore served as the untreated control group.

After 45 weeks of treatment, animals in all the three treatment regimens showed a statistically significant reduction in tumor incidence, tumor multiplicity, and tumor burden.

Note that when all the measurements were taken into consideration, namely reduction in tumor incidence, amount of tumor in grams (weight) for each tumor-bearing rat, (tumor burden) and the number

Table 7.
Effectiveness of Combined IP$_6$ + Inositol
in Mammary Tumor Model

Treatment	Tumor Incidence[1]	No. of Tumors per Rat	Rats with ≥5 Tumors, %
DMBA only	92.50% (37/40)	3.05 ± 0.35	17.5%
DMBA + IP$_6$	71.05% (27/38)[2]	2.46 ± 0.21	5.3%
DMBA + Inositol	75.00% (30/40)[2]	2.13 ± 0.2[2]	2.5%[2]
DMBA + IP$_6$ + Inositol	76.32% (29/38)[2]	1.76 ± 0.1[2]	0.0%[2]

1. Tumor incidence is shown as percentage of rats bearing a tumor divided by the total number of rats in the group as shown in parenthesis.
2. Compared to the carcinogen (DMBA)-only control group, these values are statistically significant.
Adapted from Vucenik et al., 1995.

of tumors in each tumor-bearing rat (tumor multiplicity), those animals who were treated with the combination therapy did the best; none of the animals in that group had 5 tumors. The number of tumors per rat was the lowest with the combination.

Colon cancer. Male CD-1 mice were injected with the colon carcinogen DMH (1,2-dimethylhydrazine). The drinking water of animals in the treatment groups was supplemented with either 2% inositol, or 2% IP$_6$, or 1% inositol + 1% IP$_6$. Table 8 shows the results of the experiment demonstrating the differences in results as a function of various treatments.

Table 8.
Effectiveness of IP$_6$ + Inositol in Colon Cancer Model

Experimental group	Tumor Prevalence	Tumor Frequency[a]	% Mitotic (cell division) Rate
DMH	63%[b] 12/19	22/19 (1.16)	1.92 ± 0.17
DMH + IP$_6$	47%[c] 10/21	13/21 (0.62)	1.48 ± 0.15
DMH + Inositol	30% 6/20	9/20 (0.45)	1.01 + 0.14
DMH + IP$_6$ + Inositol	25% 4/16[d]	4/16 (0.25)	1.06 + 0.13

[a]Tumor frequency is represented as number of tumors (gross + microscopic cancers) per mouse.
[b]The difference in tumor prevalence between DMH-only (carcinogen control group) and DMH + IP$_6$ + inositol[d] is significant at $p < 0.001$, and between [c]DMH + IP$_6$ and DMH + IP$_6$ + inositol at $p < 0.005$.

Thus the combination of IP$_6$ + inositol treatment is significantly better than either one alone. The results of this study showed that when all the parameters were taken into consideration, the combination therapy was the best as an anticancer regimen.

This may be a good time to summarize the results of the various studies done in animal models. The summary of the efficacy of IP$_6$ against various human and rodent, mostly human cell lines was given in Table 5 in Chapter 6. Studies from the animal experiments show that IP$_6$ and/or inositol when given either in drink or with food or injected cause significant and reproducible inhibition of the following tumor types, to date.

Table 9.
Tumors Inhibited by IP$_6$ and/or Inositol

Organ	Treatment	Mode
Colon	IP$_6$ ± ins	Drink/diet[1,2]
	inositol	Drink[1]
Fibrosarcoma	IP$_6$ ± ins	I.P[3]
	IP$_6$	Diet[4]
Liver	IP$_6$	Diet[5]
		S.C.[6]
Lungs	inositol	Diet[7]
Mammary	IP$_6$ ± ins	Drink/diet[8,9]
	inositol	Drink[8]
Muscle sarcoma	IP$_6$	S.C.[10]
Skin	IP$_6$	Drink[11]

IP$_6$ ± ins = IP$_6$ with or without inositol (ins). I.P. = intraperitoneal injection; S.C. = subcutaneous injections (for liver cancer it was intratumoral); i.e., IP$_6$ was delivered within the tumors themselves, for rhabdomyosarcoma (muscle sarcoma) it was peritumoral (around the tumor). 1. Shamsuddin et al., 1989. 2. Pretlow et al., 1992. 3. Vucenik et al., 1992. 4. Jariwalla et al., 1988. 5. Hirose et al., 1991. 6. Tantivejkul et al., 1998. 7. Wattenberg and Estensen, 1996. 8. Vucenik et al., 1995. 9. Hirose et al., 1994. 10. Vucenik et al., 1997a. 11. Zarcovic et al., 1993.

How Much to Take?

How much should we take? This depends on the reason for taking IP_6 + inositol. It can be taken as a preventative supplement for people who do not have cancer or as a dietary supplement for those who do have cancer. For a normal healthy individual, a total daily amount of 1–2 grams, or 1000–2000 milligrams, of IP_6 + inositol should be a sufficient preventative supplement to the diet. It should be taken in a divided dose, twice a day. Because of the interaction with proteins in the diet, taking it between meals would give the most optimal absorption and effectiveness. For individuals with a high risk for cancer or cardio-vascular disease, kidney stone, fatty liver, and so on, double that amount (2–4 grams per day) should be enough. And finally, for the treatment of existing cancer, the dosage will be higher—5–8 grams per day, in divided doses and between meals as previously recommended. Of course, as with any supplementation of the diet, you should consult with your health professional. I believe that in the case of existing cancer, the best use of IP_6 + inositol will be either alone or in combination with other chemotherapeutic agents to enhance effectiveness.

Epilogue

To Summarize

After reading this book, you are now familiar with the benefits of inositol and IP_6 as a potential dietary supplement. They have distinct functions and in this regard they may be considered vitamins. Inositol itself has beneficial functions against a variety of diseases such as cancer, liver diseases, neuropsychiatric disorders, and diabetes.

IP_6 is a natural antioxidant. It has an antitumor function and enhances our body's natural resistance against a variety of diseases. It also prevents kidney stones, and is responsible for a wide range of other beneficial functions by virtue of its being an antioxidant. Its beneficial function in preventing liver disease and cardiovascular disease is also important.

IP_6, however, could be seven molecules in one! By losing a phosphate group, one at a time it can be converted to $IP_{5,4,3,2,1}$ or inositol itself. The exact functions of these lower IPs are yet to be discovered, and then, who knows what we might find out about the combined benefit of the whole group? Given what we have already discovered, the possibilities are enormous. Right now, results of all the studies described in this book indicate that the combined intake of inositol + IP_6 would ensure the benefits of both of these exciting compounds and, beyond that, the synergistic effect of the formulation itself. It is a case where 1 + 1 is greater than 2!

On the Horizon: Increasing p53, a Tumor Suppressor

Some interesting developments are on the horizon. Our genetic material (the DNA) contains tumor suppressor genes. The tumor suppressor genes are so named because they are presumed to inhibit the pathways that allow the cells to become cancerous. The gene p53 acts as a molecular policeman preventing propagation of genetically damaged cells, and causes these cells to stop growing. Stopping abnormal cell growth is a right step in the direction of stopping cancer in its tracks. Mutations in the tumor suppressor genes such as p53 have been seen as contributing to the establishment of cancer. Thus, in plain terms, a normal or excess of the p53 gene is good, while mutations are bad.

Recent data from my laboratory point to the fact that IP_6 increases the expression of the tumor suppressor gene p53 by up to seventeen-fold (Saied and Shamsuddin, 1997). Along with this increased p53 expression, there was a reduction in cell proliferation and enhanced cell maturation or differentiation. As discussed earlier, more mature cancer cells are less aggressive.

The decreased expression of p53 is also associated with the resistance of tumors to chemotherapy. Thus by increasing the expression of p53, IP$_6$ is establishing its role as an adjuvant agent—one that can be used with other chemotherapeutic drugs. Standard chemotherapeutic agents have been demonstrated to be more effective if they are used in conjunction with agents that enhance p53 expression.

The World Takes Notice

The importance of IP$_6$ and inositol in the prevention and treatment of cancer and other diseases is being recognized worldwide. It is so important, in fact, that an international conference was held June 8–9, 1998. *The First International Symposium on Disease Prevention by IP-6 and Other Rice Components* at the Kyoto International Conference Hall in Kyoto, Japan, has attracted the attention of numerous scientists from around the world who have read the initial studies and are impressed. The world is taking notice; however, the U.S. medical profession has not caught up.

This symposium gathered specialists working in the field of science, research and marketing in the various industries of food, pharmaceuticals, cosmetics, and feed—for instance, rice-related agricultural education and administration—and provided them with current information on recent advances and other prospects.

The scientific program included all the topics discussed in this book:

Inositol and inositol hexaphosphate(IP_6) and its role in cellular signal transduction
Anticancer action against colon, mammary, liver and lung cancer
Protection against cardiovascular diseases
Other health benefits

Prominent amongst the speakers include George Weber, M.D., Professor and Director of the Laboratory for Experimental Oncology, Professor of Pharmacology and Milan Panic Professor of Oncology at Indiana University School of Medicine in Indianapolis. Dr. Weber has worked at the Harvard Medical School and Oxford University. He is best known for his key studies showing the differences in the biochemical strategy of normal and cancer cells. Bandaru S. Reddy, D.V.M., Ph.D., Chief, Division of Nutritional Carcinogenesis, American Health Foundation, Valhalla, New York, will also speak. Since 1995 he has been the Associate Director of the American Health Foundation. His research interests have been in the area of diet, nutrition, colon cancer, and chemoprevention of colon cancer.

Other scheduled speakers include Raxit J. Jariwalla, Ph.D., a principal research investigator in viral, immune, and metabolic diseases at the California Institute for Medical Research in San Jose. From 1982 to 1996 he was at the Linus Pauling Institute of Science and Medicine in Palo Alto, California, where he directed a program in Virology and Immunodeficiency Research, focusing studies on carcinogenesis by cancer-promoting DNA viruses and the action of antioxidants on human immunodeficiency virus. Dr. Jariwalla and his colleagues are known for their discovery of transforming genes from oncogenic human herpes viruses, identification of antitumor and lipid-lowering functions of IP_6, and the recent demonstration of suppression of HIV replication/expression by substances with antioxidant activity. Lee W. Wattenberg, Professor of Laboratory Medicine and Pathology, University of Minnesota Medical School, is called the "Father of Chemoprevention." Professor Wattenberg has championed the concept of cancer prevention by naturally occurring compounds through scientific research and by serving in many professional organizations. He was President of the American Association for Cancer Research and has received many awards for his contributions to cancer research generally.

These speakers, myself, and many others (most of whom are mentioned in this book) have striven to offer conference participants a balanced and interesting scientific program. The symposium included diverse topics ranging from cell biology, basic cancer research, clinical medicine to dietetics, organic and synthetic chemistry and biochemistry. Conference participants, scientists, and physicians themselves were able to learn and understand the wealth of research on IP_6 and inositol as you have done in reading this book. Hopefully, they will go back to their respective countries and make this information known in their medical communities.

Best of Both Worlds

Here, presented in this book, we are seeing a marriage between conventional and natural medicine. This nutritional agent, IP_6 + inositol can be used preventively, by itself, or in conjunction with chemotherapeutic drugs. This is the best of both worlds. This is the new medicine—one that uses conventional and alternative or complementary practices for the benefit of each patient. We want what works best: prevention first, treatment that is effective and safe when needed, and the ability to choose therapies that complement each other and produce the best results. This is the kind of medicine that I want for the benefit of all people. And I have dedicated my professional career and this book toward that goal.

References

Adlercreutz H, Gorbach SL, Goldin BR, Woods MN, Dwyer JT, Hämäläinen E: Estrogen metabolism and excretion in Oriental and Caucasian women. *Journal of the National Cancer Institute* 86: 1076–1082, 1994.

Agam G, Shapiro Y, Bersudsky Y, Kofman O, Belmaker RH: High-dose peripheral inositol raises brain inositol levels and reverses behavioral effects of inositol depletion by lithium. *Pharmacology, Biochemistry & Behavior* 49: 341–343, 1994.

Ames BN, Shigenaga MK, Hagen TM: Oxidants, antioxidants and the degenerative diseases of aging. *Proceedings of the National Academy of Sciences USA* 90: 7915–7922, 1993.

Arnold JT, Wilkinson BP, Sharma S, Steele VE: Evaluation of chemopreventive agents in different mechanistic classes using a rat tracheal epithelial cell culture transformation assay. *Cancer Research* 55: 537–543, 1995.

Babich H, Borenfreund E, Stern A: Comparative cyto-toxicities of selected minor dietary non-nutrients with chemopreventive properties. *Cancer Letters* 73: 127–133, 1993.

Baten A, Ullah A, Tomazic VJ, Shamsuddin AM: Inositol-phosphate-induced enhancement of natural killer cell activity correlates with tumor suppression. *Carcinogenesis* 10: 1595–1598, 1989.

Bhaskaram P, Reddy V: Role of dietary phytate in the etiology of nutritional rickets. *Indian Journal of Medical Research* 69: 265–270, 1979.

Boucher L, Chassaigne M, Ropars C: Internalization and distribution of inositol hexakisphosphate in red blood cells. *Biotechnology and Applied Biochemistry* 24: 73–78, 1996.

Burkitt DP: Epidemiology of cancer of the colon and rectum. *Cancer* 28: 3–13, 1971.

Burkitt DP: Related disease—related cause. *Lancet* 2: 1229–1231, 1969.

Challa A, Rao DR, Reddy BS: Interactive suppression of aberrant crypt foci induced by azoxymethane in rat colon by phytic acid and green tea. *Carcinogenesis* 18: 2023–2026, 1997.

Chang CS, Chen GH, Kao CH, Wang ST, Peng SN, Huang CK: The effect of *Helicobacter pylori* infection on gastric emptying of digestible and indigestible solids in patients with nonulcer dyspepsia. *American Journal of Gastroenterology* 91: 474–479, 1996.

Chung SK, Kim HH, Bahk YW: Prestenotic bronchial radioaerosol deposition: a new ventilation scan sign of bronchial obstruction. *Journal of Nuclear Medicine* 38: 71–74, 1997.

Cole KE, Smith M, Xu J-F, Vucenik I, Shamsuddin AM: Modulation of the intracellular calcium signal in human colon cancer cells by the novel anti-neoplastic agent inositol hexaphosphate. *Anticancer Research* 17: 4070, 1997.

De Stefani E, Correa P, Ronco A, Mendilaharsu M, Guidobono M, Deneo-Pellegrini H: Dietary fiber and risk of breast cancer: a case control study in Uruguay. *Nutrition and Cancer* 28: 14–19, 1997.

Dunn B: Time lag for the effect of diet on breast cancer incidence in an international study. *Proceeding of the American Association for Cancer Research* 35: 295, 1994.

Efrati Y, Horne T, Livshitz G, Broide E, Klin B, Vinograd I: Radionuclide esophageal emptying and long-acting nitrates (Nitroderm) in childhood achalasia. *Journal of Pediatric Gastroenterology & Nutrition* 23: 312–315, 1996.

Eggleton P, Penhallow J, Crawford N: Priming action of inositol hexakisphosphate (InsP$_6$) on the stimulated respiratory burst in human neutrophils, *Biochimica et Biophysica Acta* 1094: 309–316, 1991.

Estensen RD, Wattenberg LW: Studies of chemopreventive effects of *myo*-inositol on benzo[a]pyrene-induced neoplasia of the lung and forestomach of female A/J mice. *Carcinogenesis* 14: 1975–1977, 1993.

Francos RS, Barker-Gear R, Green R: Inhibition of sickling after reduction of intracellular hemoglobin concentration with an osmotic pulse: characterization of the density and hemoglobin concentration distributions. *Blood Cells* 19: 475–488, 1993, *ibid* 19: 489–491, 1993.

Fux M, Levine J, Aviv A, Belmaker RH: Inositol treatment of obsessive-compulsive disorder. *American Journal of Psychiatry* 153: 1219–1921, 1996.

Graf E, Eaton JW: Antioxidant function of phytic acid. *Free Radicals in Biology and Medicine* 8: 61–69, 1990.

Graf E, Eaton JW: Dietary suppression of colonic cancer. Fiber or phytate? *Cancer* 56: 717–718, 1985.

Graf E, Eaton JW: Effects of phytate on mineral bioavailability in mice. *J Nutr* 114: 1192–1198, 1984.

Grases F, Garcia-Ferragut L, Costa-Bauza A: A new procedure to evaluate the inhibitory capacity of calcium oxalate crystallization in whole urine. *International Urology & Nephrology* 27: 653–661, 1995.

Grases F, Garcia-Ferragut L, Costa-Bauza A: Study of the early stages of renal stone formation: experimental model using urothelium of pig urinary bladder. *Urological Research* 24: 305–311, 1996a.

Grases F, Garcia-Ferragut L, Costa-Bauza A, March JG: Study of the effects of different substances on the early stages of papillary stone formation. *Nephron* 73: 561–568, 1996b.

Harland BF, Oberleas D: Phytate in foods. *World Review of Nutrition and Diet* 52: 235–259, 1987.

Henneman PH, Benedict PH, Forbes AP, Dudley HR: Idiopathic hypercalcuria. *New England Journal of Medicine* 17: 802–807, 1958.

Hiasa Y, Kitahori Y, Marimoto J, Konishi, N, Nakaoka

S, Nishioka H: Carcinogenicity study in rats of phytic acid "Daiichi," a natural food additive. *Food and Chemical Toxicology* 30: 117–125, 1992.

Hirose M, Hoshiya T, Akagi K, Futakushi M, Ito N: Inhibition of mammary gland carcinogenesis by green tea catechins and other naturally occurring antioxidants in female Sprague-Dawley rats pretreated with 7, 12-dimethylbenz[a]anthracene. *Cancer Letters* 83: 149–156, 1994.

Hirose M, Ozaki K, Takaba K, Fukushima S, Shirai T, Ito N: Modifying effects of the naturally occurring antioxidants γ-oryzanol, phytic acid, tannic acid and n-tritriacontane-16,18-dione in rat a wide-spectrum organ carcinogenesis model. *Carcinogenesis* 12: 1917–1921, 1991.

Holub BJ: Metabolism and function of myo-inositol and inositol phospholipids. *Annual Review of Nutrition* 6: 563–597, 1986.

Huang C, Ma W-Y, Hecht SS, Dong Z: Inositol hexaphosphate inhibits cell transformation and activator protein 1 activation by targeting phosphatidylinositol-3' kinase. *Cancer Research* 57: 2873–2878, 1997.

Iqbal TH, Lewis KO, Cooper BT: Phytase activity in the human and rat small intestine. *Gut* 35: 1233–1236, 1994.

Jacobs LR: Modification of experimental colon carcinogenesis by dietary fibers. *Advances in Experimental Medicine and Biology* 206: 105–118, 1986.

Jacobs LR, Lupton JR: Relationship between colonic luminal pH, cell proliferation, and colon carcinogenesis in 1,2 dimethylhydrazine treated rats fed high fiber diets. *Cancer Research* 46: 1727–1734, 1986.

Jariwalla RJ, Sabin R, Lawson S, Bloch DA, Prender M, Andrews V, Herman ZS: Effect of dietary phytic acid (phytate) on the incidence and growth rate of tumors promoted in Fisher rats by magnesium supplement. *Nutrition Research* 8: 813–827, 1988.

Jariwalla RJ, Sabin R, Lawson S, Herman ZS: Lowering of serum cholesterol and triglycerides and modulations by dietary phytate. *Journal of Applied Nutrition* 42: 18–28, 1990.

Kamp DW, Israbian VA, Preusen SE, Zhang CX, Weitzman SA: Asbestos causes DNA strand breaks in cultured pulmonary epithelial cells: role of iron-catalyzed free radicals. *American Journal of Physiology* 268: L471–480, 1995a.

Kamp DW, Israbian VA, Yeldandi AV, Panos RJ, Graceffa P, Weitzman SA: Phytic acid, an iron chelator, attenuates pulmonary inflammation and fibrosis after intratracheal instillation of asbestos. *Toxicologic Pathology* 23: 689-695, 1995b.

Katayama T: Effect of dietary addition of *myo*-inositol on lipid metabolism in rats fed sucrose or corn starch. *Nutrition Research* 14: 699–706, 1994.

Katayama T: Effect of dietary sodium phytate on the hepatic and serum levels of lipids and on the hepatic activities of NADPH-generating enzymes in rats fed on sucrose. *Biosciences, Biotechnology and Biochemistry* 59: 1159–1160, 1995.

Kliewer EV, Smith KR: Breast cancer mortality among

immigrants in Australia and Canada. *Journal of the National Cancer Institute* 87: 1154–1161, 1995.

Kornberg A: The NIH did it! *Science* 278: 1863, 1997.

Lesser, Michael. *Nutrition and Vitamin Therapy*. New York: Bantam Books, 1981.

Levine J: Controlled trials of inositol in psychiatry. *European Neuropsychopharmacology* 7: 147–155, 1997.

Lien YH, Michaelis T, Moats RA, Ross BD: *Scyllo-inositol* depletion in hepatic encephalopathy. *Life Sciences* 54: 1507–1512, 1994.

Malhotra SL: Geographical distribution of gastrointestinal cancers in India with special reference to causation. *Gut* 8: 361–372, 1968.

Menniti FS, Oliver KG, Putney JW Jr, Shears SB: Inositol phosphates and cell signaling: new views of InsP5 and InsP6. *Trends in Biochemical Sciences* 18: 53–56, 1993.

Modlin M: Urinary phosphorylated inositols and renal stone. *The Lancet* 2(804): 1113–1114, 1980.

Nahapetian A, Young VR: Metabolism of ^{14}C-phytate in rats: effect of low and high dietary calcium intake. *Journal of Nutrition* 110: 1458–1472, 1980.

Ogawa M, Tanaka K, Kasai Z: Isolation of high phytin containing particles from rice grains using an aqueous polymer two phase system. *Agricultural Biological Chemistry* 39: 695, 1975.

Ohkawa T, Ebisuno S, Kitagawa M, Marimoto S, Miyazaki Y, Yasukawa S: Rice bran treatment for patients with hypercalciuric stones: experimental and clinical studies. *Journal of Urology* 132: 1140–1145, 1984.

Otake T, Shimonaka H, Kanai M, Miyano K, Ueba N, Kunita N, Kurimura T: Inhibitory effect of inositol hexasulfate and inositol hexaphosphoric acid (phytic acid) on the proliferation of the human immunodeficiency virus (HIV) in vitro [Japanese], *Kansenshogaku Zasshi* [Journal of Japanese Association of Infectious Diseases] 63: 676–683, 1989.

Physicians' Desk Reference Family Guide to Nutrition and Health. Montvale, NJ: Medical Economics, 1995.

Picard D, Infante-Rivard C, Villeneuve J-P, Chartrand R, Picard M, Carrier L: Extrahepatic uptake of technetium-99m-phytate: a prognostic index in patients with cirrhosis. *Journal of Nuclear Medicine* 31: 436–440, 1990.

Pretlow TP, O'Riordan MA, Pretlow TG: Colon carcinogenesis is inhibited more effectively by phytate than by selenium in F344 rats given 30 mg/kg azoxymethane. *Advances in Experimental Medicine and Biology* 354: 244, 1994.

Pretlow TP, O'Riordan MA, Somich GA, Amini SB, Pretlow TG: Aberrant crypts correlate with tumor incidence in F344 rats treated with azoxymethane and phytate. *Carcinogenesis* 13: 1509–1512, 1992.

Rao PS, Liu XK, Das DK, Weinstein GS, Tyras DH: Protection of ischemic heart from reperfusion injury by *myo*-inositol hexaphosphate, a natural antioxidant. *Annals of Thoracic Surgery* 52: 908–912, 1991.

Reddy NR, Sathe SK, Salunke DK: Phytates in legumes and cereals. *Advances in Food Research* 28: 1–89, 1982.

Reece EA, Wu Y-K: Prevention of diabetic embryopathy in offspring of diabetic rats with use of a cocktail of deficient substrates and an antioxidant. *American Journal of Obstetrics and Gynecology* 176: 790–798, 1997.

Reece EA, Eriksson UJ: The pathogenesis of diabetes-associated congenital malformations. *Obstetrics and Gynecology Clinics of North America* 23: 29–45, 1996.

Rose DP: Dietary fiber, phytoestrogens, and breast cancer. *Nutrition* 8: 47–51, 1992.

Saied IT, Shamsuddin AM: Up-regulation of the tumor suppressor gene p53 expression in HT-29 colon cancer cells by IP$_6$. *Anticancer Research* 17: 4094, 1997.

Sakamoto K, Venkatraman G, Shamsuddin AM: Growth inhibition and differentiation of HT-29 cells *in vitro* by inositol hexaphosphate (phytic acid). *Carcinogenesis* 14: 1815–1819, 1993.

Sakamoto K, Vucenik I, Shamsuddin AM: [^{3}H]Phytic acid (inositol hexaphosphate) is absorbed and distributed to various tissues in rats. *Journal of Nutrition* 123: 713–720, 1993.

Shamsuddin AM: Reduction of cell proliferation and enhancement of NK-cell activity, U. S. Patent #5 082 833: 1992.

Shamsuddin AM: A simple mucus test for cancer Screening, *Anticancer Research* 16: 2193–2200, 1996.

Shamsuddin AM, Baten A, Lalwani ND: Effect of inositol hexaphosphate on growth and differentiation in K-562 erythroleukemia cell line. *Cancer Letters* 64: 195–202, 1992.

Shamsuddin AM, Elsayed A, Ullah A: Suppression of

large intestinal cancer in F344 rats by inositol hexaphosphate. *Carcinogenesis* 9: 577–580, 1988.

Shamsuddin AM, Sakamoto K: Antineoplastic action of inositol compounds. In L. Wattenberg, M Lipkin, CW Boone and GJ Kelloff, eds. *Cancer Chemoprevention*. Boca Raton, FL C.R.C. Press, 1992, pp 285–307.

Shamsuddin AM, Ullah A: Inositol hexaphosphate inhibits large intestinal cancer in F344 rats 5 months after induction by azoxymethane. *Carcinogenesis* 10: 625–626, 1989a.

Shamsuddin AM, Ullah A, Chakravarthy A: Inositol and inositol hexaphosphate suppresses cell proliferation and tumor formation in CD-1 mice. *Carcinogenesis* 10: 1461–1463, 1989b.

Shamsuddin AM, Vucenik I, Cole KE: IP_6: A novel anticancer agent. *Life Sciences* 61: 343–354, 1997.

Shears LR, Irvine RF: Stepwise phosphorylation of myo-inositol leading to myo-inositol hexakishosphate in *Dictyostelium*. *Nature* 346: 580–583, 1990.

Shiomi S, Kuroki T, Ueda T, Takeda T, Nishiguchi S, Nakajima S, Kobayashi K, Ochi H: Diagnosis by routine scintigraphy of hepatic reticuloendothelial failure before severe liver dysfunction. *American Journal of Gastroenterology* 91: 140–142, 1996.

Subramanian G, McAfee JG, Mehter A, Blair RJ, Thomas FD: ^{99m}Tc-stannous phytate: a new in vivo colloid for imaging the reticuloendothelial system. *Journal of Nuclear Medicine* 14: 459, 1973.

Tantivejkul K, Zhang Z-S, Saied I, Vucenik I, Shamsuddin AM: Inositol hexaphosphate (IP_6) inhibits growth of human hepatocellular carcinoma. *Proceed-*

ings of American Association for Cancer Research 39: 314–315, 1998.

Thompson LU, Zhang L: Phytic acid and minerals: effect on early markers of risk for mammary and colon carcinogenesis. *Carcinogenesis* 12: 2041–2045, 1991.

Ullah A, Shamsuddin AM: Dose-dependent inhibition of large intestinal cancer by inositol hexaphosphate in F344 rats. *Carcinogenesis* 11: 2219–2222, 1990.

Unger EC, Fritz TA, Palestrant D, Meakem TJ, Granstrom P, Gatenby RA: Preliminary evaluation of iron phytate (inositol hexaphosphate) as a gastrointestinal MR contrast agent. *Journal of Magnetic Resonance Imaging* 3: 119–124, 1993.

Vucenik I, Kalebic T, Tantivejkul K, Shamsuddin AM: Inositol hexaphosphate (IP$_6$) inhibits the growth of human rhabdomyosarcoma. *Proceedings of the American Association for Cancer Research* 38: 96, 1997.

Vucenik I, Kalebic T, Tantivejkul K, Shamsuddin AM: Novel Anticancer Function of Inositol Hexaphosphate: Inhibition of Human Rhabdomyosarcoma *in vitro* and *in vivo*. *Anticancer Research,* in press.

Vucenik I, Sakamoto K, Bansal M, Shamsuddin AM: Inhibition of mammary carcinogenesis by inositol hexaphosphate (phytic acid). A pilot study. *Cancer Letters* 75: 95–102, 1993.

Vucenik I, Shamsuddin AM: [^{3}H]-Inositol hexaphosphate (phytic acid) is rapidly absorbed and metabolized by murine and human malignant cells in vitro. *Journal of Nutrition* 124: 861–868, 1994.

Vucenik I, Tomazic VJ, Fabian D, Shamsuddin AM:

Antitumor activity of phytic acid in murine transplanted and metastatic fibrosarcoma. *Cancer Letters* 65: 9–13, 1992.

Vucenik I, Yang G-Y, Shamsuddin AM: Comparison of pure inositol hexaphosphate and high-bran diet in the prevention of DMBA-induced rat mammary carcinogenesis. *Nutrition and Cancer* 28: 7–13, 1997.

Vucenik I, Yang G-Y, Shamsuddin AM: Inositol hexaphosphate and inositol inhibit DMBA-induced rat mammary cancer. *Carcinogenesis* 16: 1055–1058. 1995.

Wattenberg LW, Estensen RD: Chemopreventive effects of *myo*-inositol and dexamethasone on benzo [a]pyrene and 4-(methylnitrosoamino)-1-(3-pyridyl)-1-butanone-induced pulmonary carcinogenesis in female A/J mice. *Cancer Research* 56: 5132–5135, 1996.

Weisburger JH, Reddy BS, Rose DP, Cohen LA et al. *Basic Life Sciences* 61: 45–63, 1993.

Woolley DW: *Journal of Biological Chemistry* 139: 29–34, 1941.

Yang G-Y, Shamsuddin AM: IP_6-induced growth inhibition and differentiation of HT-29 human colon cancer cells: involvement of intracellular inositol phosphates. *Anticancer Research* 15: 2479–2488, 1995.

Zang EA, Barrett NO, Cohen LA: Differences in nutritional risk factors for breast cancer among New York City white, Hispanic, and black college students. *Ethnicity Dis* 4: 28–40, 1994.

Zaridze DG: Environmental etiology of large-bowel cancer. *Journal of the National Cancer Institute* 70: 389–400, 1983.

Zarkovic M, Nakatsuru Y, Ebina K, Ishikawa T, Shamsuddin AM: Tumor initiation inhibition by inositol hexaphosphate (InsP$_6$) in a two-stage mouse skin carcinogenesis model. *Proceedings of the Sapporo Cancer Seminar: Current Strategies of Cancer Chemoprevention*, 1993.

Zhou D-Y, Feng F-C, Zhang Y-L, Lai Z-S, Zhang W-D, Li L-B, Xu G-L, Wan T-M, Pan D-S, Zhou D, Zhang Y-C, Li S-B: Comparison of Shams' test for rectal mucus to an immunological test for fecal occult blood in large intestinal carcinoma screening. Analysis of a check-up of 6480 asymptomatic subjects. *Chinese Medical Journal* 106: 739–742, 1991.

Resources

The American Institute for Cancer Research (AICR) has provided almost $44 million for research into the role of diet and nutrition in the prevention and treatment of cancer. They provide reports on food and cancer prevention, dietary guidelines, and information on what you should be doing to achieve a lower cancer risk. AICR's free Cancer Resource cancer patient information program is available to help newly diagnosed cancer patients better understand cancer and its treatment, and to be an informed partner in fighting the disease. The Institute can be accessed on the internet at: www.aicr.org. Their mailing address is:

American Institute for Cancer Research
1759 R Street, NW
Washington, DC 20009
202-328-7744

About the Author

AbulKalam M. Shamsuddin, M.D., Ph.D., is Professor of Pathology at the University of Maryland School of Medicine in Baltimore. He teaches medical students and has been recognized as Teacher of the Year many times, most recently in 1997, by the Class of 1999.

Professor Shamsuddin graduated from Dhaka Medical College (University of Dhaka, Bangladesh) in 1972. Following his internship and residency training in Massachusetts and Maryland, he was certified by the American Board of Pathology in 1977. He received his Ph.D. in experimental pathology in 1980 at the University of Maryland, where he had joined the faculty as an instructor in 1977, rising through the ranks of assistant and associate professor, to become full professor in 1988.

Professor Shamsuddin has been studying the process of cancer formation and the prevention and therapy of cancer for the last 25 years. He has been the pioneer in discovering that inositol and inositol hexaphosphate (IP$_6$)—natural constituents of cereal grains such as rice and wheat—effectively prevent cancer formation and shrink preexisting cancers in experimental systems, with virtually no toxicity.

Professor Shamsuddin has invented several new tests for the early diagnosis and screening of colorectal cancer. One of these screening tests is called Shams' test in the Peoples' Republic of China, where it is used often. He is listed in *Who's Who of American Inventors* for his cancer screening kits.

Professor Shamsuddin has communicated the results of his research through numerous peer-reviewed papers, scientific meeting presentations, book chapters, and lectures throughout the world. He has been the principal investigator or coinvestigator for many grants from the National Cancer Institute (NCI), the American Cancer Society, and the American Institute of Cancer Research. Professor Shamsuddin has been a consultant for several NCI Review committees. As a reviewing pathologist for the Food and Drug Administration, he has evaluated suspected cancer-causing substances such as aspartame and nitrites. He has written a book for health care professionals on colon cancer screening: *Diagnostic Assays for Colon Cancer* (CRC Press, Boca Raton, Florida, 1991).